The Complete Manual on Managing Premature Ejaculation Naturally: Assurance-Based Techniques to Prolong Your Performance, Gain Complete Control, and Master Ejaculation at Will

By

Cody J. Webster

Copyright © 2023 by Cody J. Webster

The information in this book is provided for general informational purposes only and should not be construed as medical advice or instruction. Consult with a qualified healthcare professional for advice regarding your individual situation. The author and publisher make no representations or warranties with respect to the accuracy, applicability, fitness, or completeness of the contents of this book. They disclaim any warranties (expressed or implied), merchantability, or fitness for any particular purpose.

The author and publisher shall not be held liable for any loss or other damages, including but not limited to incidental, consequential, or other damages. The views expressed in this book are those of the author and do not necessarily reflect the views of the publisher.

Any resemblance to actual persons, living or dead,
or actual events is purely coincidental.

About The Author

Renowned for his extensive knowledge in the subject of sexual wellness, Cody J. Webster is a seasoned content developer. Gradually, Cody has become a well-known advocate in the field of intimate wellness, committing his time to offering thorough knowledge and advice to anyone looking to improve their sex life.

Through his work, he demonstrates his dedication to demystifying difficult sexual wellness-related subjects so that a wide range of people can grasp and relate to them. With a genuine commitment to assisting people in navigating and improving their sexual well-being, Cody's work is distinguished by a blend of in-depth research, useful ideas, and a caring attitude.

Cody's knowledge is especially deep when it comes to the complex topic of managing premature ejaculation. He enables people to extend their performance, take charge, and become proficient in ejaculation at will by using assurance-based strategies. His writing fosters a secure space for readers to explore and understand their sexual health because it is both encouraging and educational.

Cody J. Webster is an esteemed personality in the field of sexual wellness content development, and he continues to make a substantial contribution to the ongoing conversation around intimate health. His writings, which place a strong emphasis on education, dialogue, and self-empowerment, demonstrate his passion for encouraging healthy and satisfying sexual lives.

Table of Content

Introduction 11

Chapter One : Understanding Premature Ejaculation 17

Factors that Cause and Contribute 17

Psychological Aspects ... 32

Impact on Relationships and Well-Being 35

Chapter Two: Building the Foundation with Life Style Changes 39

The Importance of Leading a Healthier Lifestyle to Control Premature Ejaculation 39

Diet and Nutrition for Sexual Health 44

Cardio Workouts to Boost Endurance 48

Chapter Three: Assurance-Based Techniques for Premature Ejaculation 55

Exercises for Relaxation and Mindfulness 55

Breathing Techniques for Control 62

Visualization and Mental Conditioning 75

Chapter Four: Communication and Partner Involvement 87

Importance of Open Communication 87

Involving the Partner in the Process 99

Building a Supportive Environment 102

Chapter Five: Natural Remedies and Supplements for Premature Ejaculation 107

Medicinal Herbs for Sexual Wellness 107

Essential Nutrients and their Role 117

Add-ons to Enhance Performance 126

Chapter Six: Mastery through Practice 129

Gradual Progression in Sexual Activities 129

Methods to Postpone Ejaculation 145

Reinforcing Positive Habits 149

Chapter Seven: Overcoming Psychological Barriers in Premature Ejaculation 153

Taking Care of Performance Anxiety 153

Increasing Self-Esteem and Confidence 161

Counseling Methods for Mental Well-Being 164

Chapter Eight: Maintaining Long-Term Success 167

Strategies for Continued Improvement 167

Incorporating Techniques into Daily Life 175

Conclusions 185

Introduction

Men of all ages and backgrounds are greatly affected by premature ejaculation, or PE for short. PE, which is described by the World Health Organization as ejaculation that happens earlier than intended, affects not only the physical form but also the areas of relationships, self-worth, and general quality of life.

It happens when a man ejaculates before either he or his partner would desire. According to estimates, one in three men will experience it at some point in their lives. Though curable, PE can be an irritating and humiliating condition.

The primary indication of PE is ejaculating earlier than expected, typically two minutes after penetration or even before. From sporadic early ejaculations to a chronic pattern that interferes with sexual fulfillment, this conditions can present itself in a variety of ways.

Further signs and symptoms could be:

1. Ejaculation-induced loss of erection
2. Having trouble regulating erotic flow
3. Fear of not doing well sexually

There are many different aspects to the factors that lead to premature ejaculation, including psychological and physical aspects. PE has a variety of interrelated causes, ranging from hormone imbalances and increased penile sensitivity to performance anxiety and stress.

Recognizing the impact premature ejaculation has on people's emotional health is necessary to appreciate the seriousness of the situation. PE can worsen by creating a vicious cycle of worry due to the frustration, shame, and low self-confidence that frequently accompany the illness. This thorough review seeks to shed light on the complex aspects of early ejaculation, opening the door to a more in-depth investigation of natural, assurance-based methods that target the root reasons and enable people to find long-term solutions rather than just treating symptoms.

The case for a natural approach to treating premature ejaculation becomes more compelling in the modern world of easily accessible chemical interventions and quick solutions. A critical analysis of alternate routes to long-term sexual well-being is prompted by the drawbacks and possible adverse effects of medical remedies.

Adopting a natural approach means realizing how closely lifestyle decisions, mental health, and sexual function interact. In contrast to short-term relief from medications, a comprehensive approach tackles the underlying reasons for early ejaculation, promoting resilience and self-control over the long run.

In addition, a natural approach promotes lifestyle changes outside of the bedroom. Modifications to diet, consistent exercise, and stress reduction strategies improve general well being in addition to sexual health. The necessity of considering premature ejaculation as a comprehensive issue requiring a comprehensive and long-lasting solution—one that supports enduring vitality and is in harmony with the body's natural rhythms—is emphasized in this section of the manual.

People are urged to regain control over their sexual health by adopting a natural approach, which promotes empowerment and self-discovery. The following sections of this guide will shed light on particular lifestyle adjustments, psychological techniques, and homeopathic medicines, creating a seamless road map for achieving total control over performance and becoming proficient in ejaculation at will.

This manual sets itself apart from the plethora of self-help techniques accessible by presenting a paradigm of assurance-based approaches. In contrast to general counsel, these methods are based on a dedication to measurable outcomes, giving people a sense of assurance and confidence in their quest to stop premature ejaculation.

By providing organized, empirically supported strategies, the assurance-based approach aims to demystify the process of managing premature ejaculation. This not only creates optimism but also lays out a precise plan for reaching the intended results. By establishing a foundation of confidence in the strategies, people are inspired to begin this life-changing process with confidence in the effectiveness of the techniques offered.

This manual's upcoming sections will provide a carefully chosen collection of assurance-based methods. These methods incorporate elements of mindfulness, behavioral psychology, and holistic health, among other fields. Individuals will be guided toward mastering ejaculation at will and obtaining total control over their performance through a combination of mental conditioning, practical exercises, and lifestyle modifications.

Assurance-based therapies guarantee a profound transformation in one's connection with sexual well-being, not just an improvement. The goal as we explore the upcoming chapters is to guarantee that people will not only be able to achieve lasting control over premature ejaculation, but also to provide them with a trustworthy and efficient toolkit.

Chapter One : Understanding Premature Ejaculation

Factors that Cause and Contribute

1. Physiologic Elements

Investigating the many physiological components that lead to premature ejaculation is necessary to understand it. Developing focused therapies to manage premature ejaculation requires an understanding of how these physiological processes interact. Personalized therapy techniques are guided by the identification of individual physiological components by a full examination that includes medical history and perhaps diagnostic tests.

Now let's look at some of these factors:

1. Neurotransmitter imbalance: One neurotransmitter that is important for controlling mood and emotions is serotonin. Reduced capacity to postpone ejaculation has been linked to low serotonin levels. Sometimes doctors will prescribe drugs to correct this imbalance, such as selective

serotonin reuptake inhibitors (SSRIs), which raise
serotonin levels.

2. Glans Penis Hypersensitivity: Some people may
have the head of the penis, or the glans, more
sensitive than others. This hypersensitivity can
cause earlier arousal and ejaculation. Treatments
for this condition include topical anesthetic
desensitization or behavioral methods.

3. Genetic Predisposition: Research indicates that
premature ejaculation may have a hereditary
component. People who have a family history of
premature ejaculation may be more likely to deal
with it themselves.

4. Abnormal Reflex Activity: The ejaculatory system
may exhibit abnormal reflex activity in cases of
premature ejaculation. This might be because the
reflex pathways are more sensitive, which causes
them to react to sexual stimuli more quickly.

5. Thyroid Dysfunction: Thyroxine, in instance, is a
thyroid hormone that regulates a number of
physiological processes, including metabolism. In
addition to upsetting hormonal balance, thyroid
disease may be a factor in sexual dysfunctions such
as early ejaculation.

6. Prostate Problems: Prostatitis, or inflammation of the prostate, can affect the ability to ejaculate. Problems with the prostate may impair ejaculatory control by causing changed sensations or discomfort during sexual engagement.

7. Pelvic Floor Muscles: The ejaculatory process involves the pelvic floor muscles. Ejaculatory control may be impacted by conditions like hypertonic (overactive) or hypotonic (underactive) pelvic floor muscles. Exercises for the pelvic floor, commonly referred to as Kegel exercises, may be suggested to improve muscle tone.

8. Endocrine System Disorders: Sexual function may be impacted by endocrine system disorders, such as insufficient testosterone. For general sexual health and libido, testosterone is necessary. In cases of hormonal imbalance, hormone replacement treatment may be taken into consideration.

9. Inflammatory disorders: Discomfort and changed feelings can be caused by inflammatory disorders or infections in the urinary or genital tract, which can affect the regulation of ejaculation. In these situations, treating the underlying inflammation is crucial.

10. Peripheral Neuropathy: Damage to the peripheral nerves can result in peripheral neuropathy, which can impair motor and sensory abilities. Modified feelings and problems with ejaculation may be related to nerve injury in the genital area.

2. Physical Sensitivity

Examining the neuroanatomy, genetic influences, hormonal dynamics, psychological interactions, clinical concerns, and lifestyle factors is necessary to comprehend the complex aspects of physical sensitivity in premature ejaculation. This thorough understanding lays the groundwork for customized therapies meant to improve ejaculatory control by addressing and adjusting penile sensitivity.

1. Neuroanatomy of Penile Sensation: The penis is highly innervated, and sensory nerves are essential for sending signals pertaining to sexual desire. Genetic variations in penile sensitivity may be attributed to changes in the density and reactivity of these neurons.

2. Peripheral Nervous System Sensitivity: A person's threshold for sexual stimulation may be affected by genetic differences. A speedier

ejaculatory response may be attributed to hereditary variables that impact higher sensitivity to sexual stimulation. The peripheral nervous system's release of neurotransmitters may be influenced by genetic variables. Changes in the dynamics of neurotransmitters may impact the way signals pertaining to sexual arousal are transmitted, which could have an impact on penile sensitivity.

3. Penile Reflexes: A complicated interaction between sensory and motor neurons initiates the reflex that causes ejaculation. The effectiveness and speed of this response can be modulated by genetic factors, which can affect when a person ejaculates. Penile reflex variations may result from variations in genes linked to reflex pathways. These hereditary factors may have an impact on how quickly the ejaculatory reflex begins.

4. The Function of Hormones: Testosterone is one hormone that affects how sensitive penile tissue is. Variations in penile sensitivity among individuals may be attributed to genetic factors that impact hormone levels. Sensitivity of penile tissues to hormonal signals may be affected by genetic variations in androgen receptor genes, which are receptive to testosterone.

5. Interaction with Psychological Factors: Anxiety or arousal levels are two psychological factors that may interact with genetic predispositions for heightened penile sensitivity. This interaction can affect how arousal feels overall and raise the risk of premature ejaculation.

6. Clinical Conditions and Medications: Penile sensitivity may be affected by a number of medical illnesses, including diabetic neuropathy and neurologic abnormalities. Resolving premature ejaculation requires an understanding of and commitment to treating these underlying health conditions. Penile sensitivity may be impacted by the negative effects of some drugs, particularly those that are prescribed for other medical issues. In order to properly evaluate premature ejaculation, it is necessary to be aware of the effects of medications.

7. Genetic Predispositions: The sensitivity of dopamine and serotonin receptors may be influenced by genetic variants in these genes. The regulating function of these neurotransmitters in penile sensitivity may be impacted by altered sensitivity. Genetic influences may impact how the nervous system develops and functions, which may

have an impact on how signals pertaining to ejaculation and sexual arousal are sent.

8. Lifestyle Factors: Nutrition and food choices have an impact on neurological function as well as general health. Penile sensitivity may be impacted by nutritional imbalances or deficits. Changes in penile sensitivity may result from dehydration or health issues that impact nerve function. It is crucial to keep your body and hydration at their ideal levels.

3. Medical Issues

Understanding the impact of medical disorders on early ejaculation emphasizes the significance of a thorough medical evaluation. A comprehensive approach to controlling and enhancing ejaculatory control must address underlying health issues, whether they pertain to the prostate, thyroid, diabetes, neurological disorders, psychological conditions, or cardiovascular health.

1. Prostate Issues: Ejaculatory function may be impacted by prostatitis or other infections or inflammations of the prostate. Prostate function may be interfered with by inflammatory processes, which may lead to early ejaculation. An enlarged prostate, or benign prostatic hyperplasia (BPH),

can put pressure on the urethra and affect ejaculation. The timing of ejaculation may be affected by this physical impediment.

2. Thyroid Disorders: Hypothyroidism, or an underactive thyroid, can lower energy and metabolism. Premature ejaculation is one sexual disorder that may be caused by thyroid abnormalities.
On the other hand, hyperthyroidism, or an overactive thyroid, can cause increased metabolic rates and have an impact on sexual function. Hormonal balance can be upset by thyroid conditions, which can also affect ejaculatory regulation.

3. Diabetes: Diabetes can cause vascular problems and nerve damage (neuropathy), which can alter blood flow to the genital area. Both early ejaculation and erectile dysfunction may be caused by these issues. Diabetes has an impact on insulin resistance in particular, which affects hormone regulation. Diabetes-related hormonal abnormalities may be a factor in ejaculatory problems.

4. Neurological Disorders: Diseases such as Multiple Sclerosis (MS) can interfere with nerve signal transmission, which can impair the

coordination needed for ejaculatory regulation. Spinal cord injuries may interfere with the brain's ability to communicate with the peripheral nervous system, which could cause problems with ejaculatory function.

5. Psychiatric Disorders: Sexual function can be impacted by mental health issues, particularly anxiety and depression. Premature ejaculation may be caused by psychological variables connected to these illnesses. Sexual function may be negatively impacted by some side effects of drugs used to treat psychiatric disorders. Knowing about these possible adverse effects is essential to comprehending and controlling early ejaculation.

6. Cardiovascular Conditions: Problems with the cardiovascular system can impair blood flow to the vaginal area as well as other sections of the body. Difficulties ejaculating may be attributed to reduced blood supply. There are several drugs whose side effects affect sexual function and are prescribed for cardiovascular diseases. Recognizing these consequences is crucial for treating early ejaculation in people with cardiovascular problems.

4. Lifestyle Factors

A thorough strategy to regulating premature ejaculation must comprehend and address lifestyle issues such as food preferences, exercise routines, weight management, hydration, sleep quality, stress management, substance usage, and tobacco/nicotine intake. Changes in lifestyle can improve ejaculatory control and have a good impact on general health.

1. Diet and Nutrition: Inadequate nutrition can affect many aspects of health, including erotic activity. Certain nutrients, like omega-3 fatty acids and zinc, are important for reproductive health and may have an impact on ejaculatory regulation. Diets heavy in added sugars and processed foods can exacerbate metabolic problems and obesity. These food-related variables may affect the balance of hormones and cause early ejaculation.

2. Exercise Routines: Cardiovascular activity on a regular basis promotes better blood flow and general wellness. Sexual function depends on adequate blood circulation, and ejaculatory control may be positively impacted by cardiovascular fitness. Kegel exercises, which strengthen the pelvic floor muscles, have been shown to improve ejaculatory control. Lifestyle choices that encourage

consistent exercise, such as specific pelvic floor exercises, may be advantageous.

3. Managing Weight: Obesity is linked to a number of health problems, such as diabetes and heart disease. Premature ejaculation may result from these circumstances. For general health, maintaining a healthy weight through lifestyle decisions is crucial. Hormonal abnormalities may result from excess body fat, particularly in the belly area. Estrogen and insulin are two examples of hormones that can affect ejaculatory regulation and sexual performance.

4. Hydration: Dehydration and weariness can be caused by inadequate hydration, which can also have an adverse effect on general health. Maintaining optimal physiological function, including sexual health, requires drinking plenty of water.

5. Sleep Quality: Sleep is essential for controlling hormones, such as testosterone. Inadequate or poor quality sleep can interfere with sexual function and hormonal balance, which may lead to early ejaculation. Fatigue brought on by insufficient sleep can impair both physical and mental functioning. Ejaculatory problems may be exacerbated by

fatigue, which highlights the significance of getting enough good sleep.

6. Stress Management: Prolonged stress raises cortisol levels, which may have an effect on hormone equilibrium. Reducing the possible impact of stress on sexual function requires the use of stress management strategies, such as mindfulness and relaxation training. Premature ejaculation might be attributed to stress connected to sexual performance expectations. Effective management requires partners to communicate openly and the use of stress-reduction techniques.

7. Substance Abuse: Excessive alcohol intake and recreational drug use can affect how well the nervous system functions and can lead to problems ejaculating. Avoiding or using these substances in moderation can be advantageous.

8. Tobacco and Nicotine: These two substances have a deleterious effect on vascular health and may alter blood flow to the vaginal area. Sustaining the health of the arteries is essential for general sexual function.

5. Dynamics of Relationships

Managing and enhancing ejaculatory control requires an understanding of and attention to relationship dynamics. A good and fulfilling sexual relationship is facilitated by open communication, emotional connection, conflict resolution, sexual compatibility, and managing outside pressures. Seeking expert advice to navigate and handle certain relationship difficulties can be beneficial for couples.

1. Communication Challenges: For a sexual relationship to be healthy, effective communication regarding sexual wants, desires, and concerns is essential. Open communication about these subjects is important to avoid miscommunications and other sexual problems, such as early ejaculation. Unspoken or misinterpreted expectations about sexual performance can lead to stress and anxiety, which may affect the control of ejaculation. A harmonious sexual relationship requires that expectations are both clear and in line with one another.

2. Emotional Intimacy: Satisfaction from sex is strongly associated with emotional intimacy. Intimacy or a lack of emotional connection can aggravate sexual problems, such as early

ejaculation. Sexual well-being can be positively impacted by fortifying emotional ties. Intimate partnerships are built on trust. A lack of trust or feelings of vulnerability might affect how one feels during sexual activity. Building emotional safety and trust in the partnership is crucial.

3. Sexual Compatibility: When partners have different sexual tastes or desires, it can cause frustration and unhappiness. A satisfying sexual relationship requires addressing and compromising on sexual compatibility. A healthy sexual relationship can be facilitated by being willing to experiment with and accommodate each other's sexual inclinations. A more fulfilling sexual relationship is cultivated via open communication and experimentation.

4. Unresolved Issues: Relationship stress or unresolved problems can sometimes find their way into the bedroom. A harmonious sexual relationship requires cooperatively addressing and resolving issues. Conflict-related emotional fallout can provide a bad environment that may affect sexual intimacy. It's critical to identify healthy strategies for addressing and releasing emotional stress.

5. Intimacy Outside the Bedroom: Providing emotional support to a partner outside of a sexual setting enhances their contentment in the relationship as a whole. An atmosphere of support fosters emotional intimacy, which improves sexual well-being. Connections are forged via shared hobbies and meaningful time spent together. Building a solid foundation outside of the bedroom can have a beneficial impact on sexual dynamics.

6. External Stressors: Experiencing financial hardships can lead to stress that seeps into every area of life, including relationships. It's critical to reduce financial stress by working together to solve problems and communicate effectively. Parenting responsibilities might affect intimacy. A successful sexual relationship requires striking a balance between raising children and preserving a love bond.

7. Cultural and Religious Influences: Expectations regarding sexual behavior might be influenced by cultural or religious beliefs. Disparities in these expectations between couples may be a factor in communication and sexual dysfunction. It is crucial to comprehend and honor cultural or religious variations around sexuality. An honest discussion

about these disparities encourages acceptance and understanding between people.

Psychological Aspects

Understanding the complex interaction between psychological elements that contribute to premature ejaculation is crucial for a holistic therapy strategy. A comprehensive approach to enhance ejaculatory control must address prior trauma, manage stress, cultivate good relationship dynamics, promote positive self-image, address performance anxiety, and take depression into account. A more successful and long-lasting strategy benefits from teamwork between individuals and their partners as well as professional support when required.

1. Performance anxiety: The worry of falling short of perceived standards during sexual engagement is known as performance anxiety and is a prevalent psychological element in premature ejaculation. A self-fulfilling prophesy is created by this fear of failing because anxiety can lead to early ejaculation. People who are anxious about performing may start thinking negatively about their sexual prowess. Premature ejaculation might be perpetuated by a

cycle of worry triggered by these ideas. The goal of cognitive-behavioral techniques is to confront and alter these unfavorable thought habits.

2. Stress and Cortisol Levels: Prolonged stress triggers the release of cortisol as a result of the body's stress response. High cortisol levels have the potential to cause premature ejaculation by upsetting hormonal balance and severely affecting sexual performance. Cortisol production brought on by stress may disrupt the physiological mechanisms governing sexual arousal and responsiveness. Reducing stress and its negative effects on sex performance requires practicing mindfulness and relaxation techniques.

3. Relationship Dynamics: Emotional distance and misplaced expectations can result from partners' inability to freely communicate sexual difficulties with one another. Premature ejaculation may persist as a result of this communication breakdown. Sexual happiness in a relationship is strongly impacted by the level of emotional connection. Unresolved issues or insufficient emotional connection might act as a psychological barrier that interferes with ejaculatory control.

4. Body Image and Self-Esteem: Feelings of inadequacy during sexual encounters can be caused by poor body image and low self-esteem. People who have a negative body image could be more likely to experience performance anxiety, which could lead to early ejaculation.
A healthy sexual mindset requires both sexual confidence and a positive self-image. Enhancing sexual confidence and self-worth can help mitigate the psychological effects of early ejaculation.

5. Past Trauma or Abuse: Sexual function may be significantly impacted psychologically by past trauma or abuse experiences. Intimate times might bring up painful memories, which can lead to early ejaculation. Therapy that focuses on trauma is essential for resolving these underlying problems. Establishing emotional safety and trust is crucial for people who have experienced trauma in the past. Creating a safe space is critical to breaking through the psychological barriers brought up by traumatic experiences.

6. Depression and Libido: Depression can affect arousal and ejaculatory control, as well as result in a decreased interest in sex. Depression's neurochemical and psychological components may play a role in early ejaculation.

Although antidepressant drugs treat depression, they may have adverse consequences on a person's ability to conceive. Managing premature ejaculation in individuals with depression requires striking a balance between mental health treatment and knowledge of potential negative effects.

Impact on Relationships and Well-Being

Premature ejaculation is linked to emotional health and interpersonal dynamics, which highlights the necessity for a comprehensive management strategy. This entails having honest conversations, supporting one another, dealing with problems related to one's self-worth, and, if need, obtaining professional help. Individuals and their partners can effectively negotiate the problems presented by premature ejaculation by exercising empathy, understanding, and a collaborative approach, while also taking into account the broader impact on relationships and overall well-being.

1. Communication Issues: Early ejaculation can cause a breakdown in communication between partners because the person experiencing it may be reluctant or ashamed to talk about it honestly. This communication breakdown can cause a rift, making

it impossible for the couple to work together to solve the issue. The affected person could find it difficult to communicate their sexual demands or talk about the difficulties they are having. The couple's capacity to cooperate to find a solution may be hampered by this quiet, which may cause miscommunication.

2. Emotional Disturbances: Prolonged problems with early ejaculation may be a factor in the development of emotional distancing between partners. The condition's related frustrations and disappointments might act as a barrier, reducing the emotional connection that is essential to a happy and fulfilling relationship. Physical intimacy can result from emotional distance, which can impact the relationship's overall quality. Both spouses may feel alone as a result of the absence of intimacy.

3. Diminished Self-Esteem: Premature ejaculation can have a substantial negative effect on a person's self-esteem. Persistent experiences of feeling inadequate sexually can result in a negative self-perception and decreased self-assurance, which can impact different facets of their life. The partner might also feel worried or frustrated, which could cause them to struggle emotionally. Experiencing a

loved one battle with low self-esteem can be emotionally draining and negatively impact both parties' general wellbeing.

4. Sexual Satisfaction: Both partners may experience less sexual satisfaction if premature ejaculation is a recurring occurrence. This discontent could start a vicious cycle of avoiding or being reluctant to have sex, which would strain the relationship even more. The general quality of a relationship is strongly correlated with sexual satisfaction. Sexual problems can have a domino effect on how a couple views their relationship, which could result in discontent in other areas as well.

5. Implications for Mental Health: For the person undergoing the disease, premature ejaculation may lead to increased tension, anxiety, or even depressive symptoms. These effects on daily functioning and general well-being are not limited to the bedroom. Premature ejaculation-related mental health issues might affect how partners communicate and encourage one another. Establishing a supportive environment requires an understanding of these issues and solutions.

6. Working Together to Find Solutions: Collaboratively addressing the effects of early ejaculation on relationships and overall health is possible when this issue is acknowledged. Collaboratively addressing the emotional toll of the disease increases the likelihood of relationship strengthening and successful problem solving for couples. The emotional and relational fallout from early ejaculation can be addressed in a structured and encouraging setting by seeking professional assistance, such as through couples therapy or sex therapy. Professional interventions could involve exercises in emotional connection, communication techniques, and coping skills for both parties.

Chapter Two: Building the Foundation with Life Style Changes

Using a comprehensive strategy is necessary to provide the groundwork for better sexual health through lifestyle modifications. Ejaculatory control can be positively impacted by leading a healthy lifestyle that includes stress management, frequent exercise, and a nutritious diet. Comprehensive efforts to manage premature ejaculation and promote a healthier and more enjoyable sexual experience are based on these lifestyle modifications.

The Importance of Leading a Healthier Lifestyle to Control Premature Ejaculation

Living a healthy lifestyle is essential to preserving general health and having a good quality of life. It includes a range of elements, such as mental, emotional, and physical health. Healthy lifestyle choices can lower the chance of developing chronic illnesses, increase mental acuity and emotional stability, and boost vitality in general.

Benefits of a healthy lifestyle for mental, emotional, and physical health:

1. Decreased risk of chronic illnesses: Leading a healthy lifestyle can dramatically reduce your chance of contracting long-term illnesses like heart disease, stroke, type 2 diabetes, and some cancers.

2. Better weight management: It's critical for general health to maintain a healthy weight with a balanced diet and frequent exercise. It lowers the chance of obesity and the health issues that go along with it.

3. Improved physical fitness: Engaging in regular exercise increases endurance, strengthens bones and muscles, and improves cardiovascular health.

4. Less Stress and Anxiety: Stress levels and anxiety can be efficiently managed with the help of good habits like consistent exercise, enough sleep, and relaxation techniques. Prolonged stress is frequently linked to early ejaculation.

Ejaculatory control can be favorably impacted by leading a healthy lifestyle that incorporates stress-reduction practices like deep breathing exercises and meditation. Cortisol is released in response to stress, which can throw off the balance of hormones. Cortisol levels are regulated by a healthy lifestyle that includes good stress management, which lessens the possibility of its detrimental effects on sexual performance.

5. Better mood and cognitive performance: Living a healthy lifestyle contributes to mental health, which in turn improves mood, concentration, and cognitive performance.

6. Greater Emotional Well-Being and Resilience: Developing positive habits can improve emotional resilience, which helps people deal with life's obstacles and stay emotionally stable. Anxiety and performance-related stress are two psychological variables that lead to early ejaculation.
These psychological issues can be lessened by leading a healthy lifestyle that promotes mental resilience through constructive behaviors and stress-reduction strategies.

7. Promotes Hormonal Balance: Hormones are essential for maintaining sexual health, which includes controlling ejaculation. Better sexual function is supported by a healthy lifestyle that includes regular exercise and a balanced diet, which supports hormonal balance. The hormone

testosterone, which is important for male sexual health, is impacted by lifestyle choices. Sufficient sleep, consistent exercise, and a healthy diet all help to keep testosterone levels at their ideal levels, which can have a beneficial effect on ejaculatory control.

8. Cardiovascular Health: Poor blood flow to the genital area is frequently linked to premature ejaculation. A healthy lifestyle includes cardiovascular activity, which enhances blood circulation generally and supports ejaculatory control and erectile performance. Vascular integrity is maintained by a healthy cardiovascular system, which guarantees that blood vessels operate at their best. Maintaining the physiological mechanisms involved in sexual response requires this.

9. Neurological well-being: Living a healthy lifestyle influences the way the neural system that controls sexual response functions. A nutrient-rich diet and regular exercise promote proper neurological function, which may help with ejaculatory regulation.

10. Strength of the Pelvic Floor Muscles: The regulation of ejaculation is influenced by the Pelvic Floor muscles. To strengthen these muscles and

maybe improve ejaculatory control, a healthy lifestyle routine should include specific exercises like Kegels that target the pelvic floor. In order to effectively manage premature ejaculation, physical factors such as the strength of the pelvic floor muscles must be addressed. This comprehensive approach includes regular exercise, including pelvic floor exercises.

11. General Physical Fitness: An individual's endurance and stamina during sexual engagement can have an impact on premature ejaculation. Frequent exercise increases physical fitness overall, increases endurance and stamina, and enhances sexual performance. Energy levels are raised by a balanced diet and regular exercise in a healthy lifestyle. During sexual experiences, increased energy translates to enhanced vitality, potentially positively

12. Relationship dynamics and emotional well-being are positively impacted by a healthy lifestyle, which promotes emotional well-being. Stressors associated with premature ejaculation may be reduced in a relationship by open communication, mutual support, and shared activities. Relationship tension might arise from premature ejaculation. This stress can be reduced

by leading a healthy lifestyle that incorporates relationship-building and emotional well-being techniques, creating a caring and understanding environment.

Diet and Nutrition for Sexual Health

A healthy, well-balanced diet is essential for preserving sexual function and health. Vitamins, minerals, and antioxidants are examples of essential nutrients that support healthy reproductive organs, appropriate hormone production, and general energy levels. For sexual health, including ejaculatory control, a diet high in vital nutrients that promote hormonal balance, vascular health, and general well-being is needed. Incorporating complete, unprocessed foods, drinking enough of water, and limiting alcohol use are all parts of a comprehensive nutrition strategy that enhances sexual performance and promotes a healthy way of life.

1. Diet High in Nutrients Hormonal equilibrium, which is crucial for sexual health, can only be preserved by eating a diet high in nutrients. Zinc is a nutrient that is essential for the creation of testosterone, which affects ejaculatory control and sexual function. Nuts like zinc are present in foods

like lean meats and nuts. Higher levels of vitamin D are linked to better reproductive health. Sunlight exposure, fortified dairy products, and fatty seafood are good sources of vitamin D. A healthy level of vitamin D is linked to general sexual health. Walnuts, flaxseeds, and seafood are good sources of omega-3 fatty acids, which are important for neurotransmitter activity. Serotonin and other neurotransmitters possibly play a role in controlling sexual response.

2. Blood Flow and Vascular Health: Sexual function, including the erection and ejaculatory processes, depends on adequate blood circulation. Berries, leafy greens, and whole grains are among the foods that maintain healthy blood flow to the genital area and promote vascular health. Foods like garlic and beets help produce nitric oxide, which is a chemical that aids in blood vessel dilatation. Higher nitric oxide levels have a beneficial effect on blood flow, which may improve sexual function.

3. Hydration: Staying well hydrated is essential for good health in general and for healthy sexual performance in particular. Fatigue and low energy levels brought on by dehydration may have an impact on sexual performance. The health of

mucous membranes, particularly those in the genital area, is supported by hydration. Mucous membranes that are properly hydrated help to make sexual action more comfortable.

4. Reducing Processed Foods and Sugars: Obesity is associated with diets heavy in processed foods and added sugars, which can upset the hormonal balance. Eating complete, unprocessed foods to maintain a healthy weight promotes hormonal balance, which has a favorable impact on sexual health. Processed meals frequently cause inflammation, which has a detrimental effect on vascular health and blood flow. Selecting entire meals that have anti-inflammatory qualities, such fruits and vegetables, promotes healthy sexual functioning in general.

5. Moderate Alcohol Consumption: Drinking too much alcohol might damage the nerve system, which can impact one's ability to mate. Consuming alcohol in moderation supports healthy nervous system function, which may have a beneficial effect on ejaculatory regulation. Because alcohol dehydrates the body, it can exacerbate weariness. Drinking alcohol in moderation and staying well-hydrated help to minimize any potential harm to one's energy and sexual performance.

Essential nutrients for healthy sexual function:

Zinc: Zinc promotes healthy sperm production and is necessary for males to produce testosterone.

Vitamin D: Vitamin D is important for libido regulation and sexual function maintenance.

Folate: Preventing birth abnormalities and preserving the health of reproductive organs depend on folate.

Iron: Low energy and decreased libido might result from an iron deficit.

Omega-3 fatty acids: These fats lower inflammation and help produce hormones, both of which can lead to sexual dysfunction.

Dietary guidelines for maintaining sexual health: Eat a range of fruits, vegetables, and whole grains. These foods are rich in antioxidants, vitamins, and minerals that are necessary for maintaining sexual health.

Add sources of lean protein: The essential amino acids required for hormone production and tissue repair are found in lean protein sources such as fish, poultry, and beans.

Select good fats like nuts, seeds, and avocados are rich sources of healthy fats that promote hormone production and lower inflammation.

Reduce your intake of processed meals, sugar-filled beverages, and excessive alcohol as sexual function and hormone balance may be adversely affected by these.

Exercise Routines for Improved Stamina

Engaging in consistent physical exercise is crucial for boosting general vitality and endurance. Exercises that combine cardiovascular and weight training can significantly improve stamina and endurance.

Cardio workouts to boost endurance:

- Running: Enhancing cardiovascular health, endurance, and stamina, running is a great cardio workout.

- Swimming is a low-impact aerobic workout that increases muscular strength and general fitness.

- Riding a bicycle is a fantastic way to enjoy the outdoors and increase stamina and endurance.

Benefits:

1. Increased Cardiovascular Health through Cardiovascular Exercise: Cardiovascular health is enhanced by regular cardiovascular exercise, such as swimming, cycling, or jogging. Better blood circulation is facilitated by improved heart and lung function, which supplies essential oxygen and nutrients to the muscles used in sexual activity.

Endurance and stamina are strongly related to cardiovascular fitness. Regular cardiovascular exercisers frequently report increased physical stamina, which has a favorable effect on their capacity to maintain sexual engagement.
The genital area receives excellent blood flow when one engages in cardiovascular exercise. This improved blood flow can have a beneficial effect on ejaculatory control and is necessary for erectile function.

2. Pelvic Floor Exercises: Also referred to as Kegels, these exercises target and strengthen the muscles that are part of the ejaculatory reflex. Better control over the timing of ejaculation may result from increased tone in the pelvic floor muscles. Exercises for the pelvic floor are a component of a holistic strategy for sexual wellness. They improve ejaculatory control and overall performance by targeting particular muscle areas related to sexual function.

3. Strength Training: Weightlifting and resistance training are examples of strength training exercises that improve muscle tone and endurance. Stronger muscles contribute to greater physical endurance, which enhances sexual performance.
One essential element of overall physical fitness is strength training.

Strength training is a part of a well-rounded fitness regimen that helps to boost vitality and energy, both of which are important for sexual health. Hormonal balance can be positively impacted by strength exercise. Exercise causes the release of endorphins, which improve mood and may mitigate the effects of stress by promoting hormonal balance.

4. Mind-Body and Yoga Practices: Mind-body therapies, like yoga and meditation, are useful for lowering anxiety and stress levels. Premature ejaculation is frequently caused by stress, thus lowering stress levels using these techniques can have a favorable effect on ejaculatory control. Yoga encourages relaxation and an awareness of one's bodily feelings by fostering a mind-body connection. This increased consciousness may also apply to sexual encounters, thereby improving general sexual health. The practises of yoga and meditation help to enhance mental health. Positivity enhances sexual performance and may have a beneficial effect on ejaculatory control.

5. Consistency and Variety: People are more likely to maintain their fitness regimens when they engage in regular, varied workout routines that avoid boredom. Frequent exercise improves energy, lowers stress, and increases stamina, all of which are beneficial for improved sexual performance. Consistent work is necessary for long-term gains in physical fitness.

Frequent exercise has extensive advantages for general health and sexual function, including cardiovascular, strength training, and mind-body techniques. Strength training, aerobic activity, pelvic floor exercises, and mind-body techniques all work together to improve sexual health and stamina in a comprehensive way. Each element works in concert with the others to improve both physical and mental health.

Strengthening workouts to improve endurance:

Squats: Squats improve the strength of the lower body muscles, which are essential for general endurance and stamina.

Lunges: Lunges strengthen the muscles in the legs and boost balance, which can help with stamina and athletic performance.

Push-ups: These exercises build the muscles in the upper body, which enhances general strength and stamina.

Other advice for enhancing endurance:

Start out slowly and lengthen the duration and intensity gradually. Repercussions and injuries might result from overexertion.

When necessary, pay attention to your body and take days off. Rest stops overtraining and enables muscles to repair.

Drink plenty of water: Staying well hydrated is crucial for both general health and peak performance during exercise.

Keep up a healthy diet: Energy and nutrients needed to promote endurance and stamina are found in a balanced diet.

A balanced diet, consistent exercise, and enough sleep are all important components of a healthy lifestyle that will sustain general wellbeing, improve sexual health, and increase stamina. People can greatly enhance their physical, mental, and emotional well-being and live happier, more satisfying lives by adopting good habits and making deliberate decisions.

Chapter Three: Assurance-Based Techniques for Premature Ejaculation

Exercises for Relaxation and Mindfulness

1. Awareness in the Context of Sexuality

Deep, deliberate breaths are taken and released as part of the mindfulness and relaxation practice of mindful breathing. In order to promote a more relaxed and alert state of mind, this practice invites people to concentrate on their breathing. Mindful breathing can be used to reduce anxiety, maintain present-moment awareness, and promote calm mental states in sexual encounters. Anyone looking to improve control over their ejaculation and develop a more laid-back attitude toward sexual encounters would find this practice beneficial.

To improve relaxation and encourage a more controlled and pleasurable approach to sexual performance, techniques such as guided visualization and focused breathing are applied.

2. The progressive relaxation of muscles (PMR)

A systematic method called Progressive Muscle Relaxation (PMR) includes consciously tensing and then relaxing various bodily muscle groups. PMR is used as a mindfulness and relaxation technique to ease stress, lessen anxiety, and foster a general sense of calm. When it comes to sexual encounters, PMR can be a useful technique for people who want to improve their ability to regulate their erection and adopt a more optimistic outlook. Muscle Relaxation (PMR) is an effective mindfulness and relaxation technique that provides people with a methodical way to ease tension and anxiety. When used in the context of sexual encounters, PMR can support a more relaxed and controlled approach, which may improve general sexual well-being and ejaculatory control. Consistent application and incorporation into one routine are key to unlocking the full benefits of this mindfulness technique.

Elements of PMR:

1. Guided Tension and Release: PMR is usually conducted under guidance, taking the patient through a series of muscle groups. This might begin from the toes and work its way up, or it could take a different path, gradually working on various body

parts. To start the workout, consciously tense a certain muscle group. This stage increases awareness of tense muscles and gets the person ready for the next relaxation.
People are told to fully release their tension after tensing up so that their muscles can relax. The targeted muscle areas experience deep relaxation during this phase.

2. Awareness and Mind-Body Connection: People who practice PMR are encouraged to concentrate on the bodily sensations connected to both relaxation and tension. A key component of mindfulness is the mind-body connection, which is fostered by this increased awareness. Each muscle group's minute distinctions between tension and relaxation are pointed out to participants. This sensory awareness enhances the technique's overall efficacy.

3. Application to Sexual Context: PMR can lessen anxiety associated to performance when it comes to sexual encounters. People who regularly release their tense muscles may feel more at ease and in control, which can help reduce the risk of premature ejaculation. PMR heightens awareness of physical feelings, which is especially advantageous in intimate situations. People are able

to remain mindful of their body and stay in the present moment because of this increased awareness.

4. Integration into Routine: Consistent practice is advised to optimize PMR's advantages. Regular practice of this mindfulness exercise helps people become more adept at bringing themselves into a relaxed state, which makes it easier to access during sex. People are able to include PMR into their pre-sexual practices. This proactive strategy encourages a calm frame of mind, which may lessen performance anxiety and assist ejaculatory control.

Advantages of PMR for Relaxation and Mindfulness:

By encouraging relaxation throughout the body, PMR is useful in lowering overall stress levels. Regular PMR practice has also been linked to better sleep, which enhances general wellbeing.

By promoting mental calmness, PMR can assist people in controlling their emotions.

PMR cultivates a heightened awareness that can enhance focus and concentration, both of which are beneficial in intimate situations.

3. Guided Imagery

Using vivid mental images to encourage relaxation, lower stress levels, and improve general well-being, guided imagery is a mindfulness and relaxation practice. Guided imagery can be an effective method for people who want to regulate their nervousness, enhance their ability to ejaculate, and cultivate a pleasant mental state when it comes to sexual experiences.

As a useful mindfulness and relaxation technique, guided imagery gives people a way to de-stress and build a happy mental environment. When used in conjunction with sexual encounters, guided imagery can help promote a more laid-back attitude and possibly enhance

Essential Elements of Guided Imagery:

1. Visualization Techniques: The first step in guided imagery is to form precise mental images. These visuals, which concentrate on situations or locations that arouse feelings of serenity, enjoyment, and good vibes, are frequently self-directed or directed by a narrator. Multiple senses are stimulated by effective guided visualization. It is suggested that people picture the scene as well as fully immerse themselves in the sound, smell, and touch elements.

2. Narration and Guidance: External guidance is a common feature of guided imagery sessions. This direction can be from self-directed meditation apps, a live facilitator, or an audio script that has been produced. The person is guided through the visualizing process by the guide. A soothing, tranquil tone is frequently employed by narrators to augment the relaxation reaction. This tone helps the person establish a secure and peaceful mental environment.

3. Application to Sexual Context: Positive sexual situations might be included in guided imagery while discussing sexual experiences. People can see themselves in happy, fulfilling scenarios, which helps them associate having sex with positive things. By shifting attention away from possible stresses and onto uplifting and joyful mental images, guided imagery can help lessen anxiety associated to performance. This change in focus leads to a more at ease mood.

Guided imagery is frequently most effective with regular practice to optimize the advantages. People can become proficient at using this approach as a relaxing tool by engaging in it consistently. It might be very helpful to incorporate guided visualization into pre-sexual rituals. By practicing mindfulness before intimate situations, you can create a nice atmosphere and possibly enhance your general sexual health.

The advantages of guided imagery for relaxation and mindfulness

The benefits of guided imagery in lowering stress and encouraging a state of mental and physical relaxation are well-established.

Guided imagery is a technique for emotional regulation that helps people manage their anxiety and negative emotions by focusing the mind on peaceful and positive pictures.

Frequent use of guided imagery helps people have a more optimistic view on life in general and certain circumstances in particular, including sexual encounters.

The concentrated attention needed for guided imagery sessions improves mental focus and concentration, which may have a positive impact on mental health in general.

Breathing Techniques for Control

Deep Diaphragmatic Breathing
One of the most effective breathing techniques for controlling anxiety, enhancing control over physiological responses, and promoting relaxation is deep diaphragmatic breathing, particularly during sexual activity. Through deliberate, leisurely inhalation and exhalation, the diaphragm is engaged, resulting in a deeper, more peaceful breathing cycle.

During sexual activity, deep diaphragmatic breathing is an effective breathing technique that can help with control, anxiety management, and relaxation. Through persistent practice and integration of this strategy into pre-sexual rituals, people can optimize their general sexual well-being and ejaculatory control.

Its elements includes:

1. Diaphragmatic Engagement: The diaphragm, a sizable muscle situated between the chest and abdomen, is the main target of this exercise. The diaphragm contracts during inhalation, enabling the lungs to expand and take in air. Exhalation entails the diaphragm relaxing. When

diaphragmatic breathing occurs, the abdomen frequently moves visibly. The belly expands on breath and collapses on exhalation when the diaphragm contracts.

2. Slow and Controlled Breathing: The emphasis of deep diaphragmatic breathing is on breathing at a slower, more deliberate pace. People can take a breath, hold it for a moment, and then let out a somewhat longer breath. The nervous system is calmed by reducing the pace of breathing. This deliberate pacing helps manage arousal levels, contributing to better control during intimate moments.

3. Concentrate on Breath Awareness: By focusing on the breath, deep diaphragmatic breathing integrates awareness. People concentrate on the feeling of air coming into and going out of their bodies, which promotes a mindful and in-the-moment attitude. Focusing on the breath might help people refocus their attention from worries about sexual performance that cause anxiety. This diversion helps to promote a calmer state of mind.

4. During sexual engagement, deep diaphragmatic breathing is very helpful in controlling arousal

levels. People can avoid the fast breathing patterns linked to increased arousal by practicing calm breathing. Anxiety associated to performance can be effectively managed using this breathing method. Deep diaphragmatic breathing has a relaxing impact that supports ejaculatory control by creating a positive mental space.

5. One way to prepare for sexual activity before engaging in it is to practice deep diaphragmatic breathing. This proactive strategy creates a laid-back atmosphere that facilitates improved control. Incorporating deep diaphragmatic breathing into one's habit requires regular practice. Maintaining consistency enables people to become accustomed to the method, which makes it easier to use when tension or anxiety levels are high.

Advantages of Controlling Deep Diaphragmatic Breathing:

By inducing the relaxation response, deep diaphragmatic breathing lowers general stress levels and fosters mental clarity.

This method guarantees that the body receives the ideal amount of oxygen, promoting physiological functions and general health.

Breathing with the diaphragm activates respiratory efficiency and helps create a more regulated and controlled breathing rhythm.

Paying mindful attention to one's breathing promotes better focus and concentration, which is advantageous in private situations.

The 4-7-8 Method for Controlled Breathing
A particular breathing exercise called the 4-7-8 technique is intended to help with relaxation, breathing pattern regulation, and improving control over physiological responses. With this technique, breath-holding, inhalation, and exhalation are done in a prescribed order and for a predetermined number of counts. This deliberate breathing pattern is known to have a calming effect on the nervous system and may help with improved control in a variety of settings, including private ones.
The 4-7-8 technique is a useful breathing exercise that improves control over physiological responses, promotes relaxation, and regulates breathing patterns. Because of its methodical flow, it's a useful tool for people who want to reduce their stress and anxiety, especially in situations where it's beneficial to breathe deliberately, as during intimate times. Regular practice and integration

into routine rituals contribute to maximizing the benefits of this breathing technique.

Elements of the 4-7-8 Method:

1. The Structured Breathing Sequence:

- Four counts of inhalation People start by taking a slow, deep breath through their nostrils while counting to four. This deliberate inhalation establishes the rhythm throughout the entire sequence and aids in oxygenation of the lungs.

- Holding the Breath for Seven Counts: After taking a breath, people hold it for seven counts. The nervous system is calmed and oxygen is better absorbed during this little break.

- Exhaling for Eight Counts: When exhaling, the breath is slowly and deliberately released through the mouth for eight counts. This long exhale helps clear the lungs of stagnant air and encourages calm.

2. Nervous System and Breathing Regulation:
The 4-7-8 technique's systematic approach activates the parasympathetic nerve system, which

is commonly known as the "rest and digest" system. Switching on this system helps promote a relaxed and tranquil frame of mind.

The breathing pattern is controlled by the deliberate counts made during inhalation, breath-holding, and exhale. The fast, shallow breathing linked to tension and anxiety can be countered by this rhythmic breathing.

3. The 4-7-8 approach works especially well in situations where controlling arousal is required, such as during sexual encounters. An intentional breath-holding phase and a prolonged exhale help to regulate the body's reaction more tightly. People can refocus their attention from performance-related worry to the rhythmic and relaxing process of breathing by using this structured breathing routine. A more at ease mental state is supported by this change in focus.

4. It may be helpful to incorporate the 4-7-8 approach into pre-sexual rituals. Setting a calm and positive atmosphere for intimate encounters can be achieved by practicing this breathing technique beforehand. The 4-7-8 technique is more effective with repeated practice, just like many other breathing techniques. Regular participation enables

people to become accustomed to the sequence, making it easier to understand during moment of stress.

Advantages of the 4-7-8 Control Method:

Stress levels are swiftly lowered by the systematic breathing pattern, which triggers a relaxation reaction.

The intentional breathing and holding of the breath phases maximize the absorption of oxygen, promoting general health.

The 4-7-8 approach promotes mindfulness and present-moment awareness, which enhances concentration and focus.

Heart rate and blood pressure are two physiological responses that are calmed by a regular breathing pattern.

Coordinated Breathing with a Partner
Synchronized breath patterns during sexual activity are a part of the collaborative and personal practice of coordinated breathing with a partner. In addition to fortifying the emotional bond between lovers, this shared experience helps to maintain a more

controlled and mutually satisfying sexual experience by managing arousal levels.

A relevant and useful technique that improves the emotional and physical components of a sexual relationship is coordinated breathing with a partner. By breathing in unison, the two people establish a common rhythm that promotes relaxation, arousal control, and a stronger sense of connection. As with any personal practice, the foundation of a happy relationship is open communication and a readiness to discover and accommodate one another's preferences.

The important aspects include:

1. Breathing Synchronization: Partners match the depth and rate of their breaths by synchronizing their breathing patterns. In private moments, this fosters a sense of oneness and shared experience. It takes deliberate effort to synchronize the inhale and exhale during the practice. A particular rhythm that is easy and natural for both parties can be selected by partners.

2. Emotional Bonding: Intimacy between spouses is enhanced by coordinated breathing. The shared breath fosters emotional intimacy by establishing a nonverbal bond that goes beyond words.

Coordinated breathing builds a stronger bond and a sense of shared awareness between partners by encouraging them to be present with one another in the moment.

3. Reciprocal Arousal Control: By calming both lovers, synchronized breathing can help with reciprocal arousal control. Heart rate and tension are two physiological responses that are regulated by the coordinated rhythm. Couples might potentially reduce performance anxiety and create a more comfortable environment for sexual engagement by participating in synchronized breathing exercises together.

4. Communication and Trust: One way to communicate nonverbally is to breathe in unison. Without using words, it enables partners to communicate their connection and attunement. Coordination of breathing exercises fosters vulnerability and trust in relationships. This vulnerability on both sides can improve the quality of the sexual relationship as a whole.

5. Intimate moments are smoothly infused with coordinated breathing. It develops into an organic and intuitive aspect of the sexual encounter, fostering a healthy bond. Depending on their tastes,

partners might alter their coordinated breathing technique. This method's adaptability enables modifications to meet each person's comfort level and preferences.

Advantages of Partner-Coordinated Breathing for Control:

Coordinated breathing strengthens the emotional relationship between partners and fosters a deeper, more meaningful connection.

During sexual action, coordinated breathing helps to create a relaxed and pleasant environment by encouraging a sense of mutual relaxation.

In order to create a more mutually happy sexual experience, the practice synchronizes arousal levels between couples.

A sense of unity and attentiveness is promoted by coordinated breathing, which acts as a nonverbal communication of intimacy.

Box Breathing for Breathing Control
Also referred to as square breathing, box breathing is a controlled breathing method that entails taking a breath, holding it for a set amount of time,

releasing, and then holding it again. Since it produces a balanced and rhythmic breathing pattern, this technique is useful for people who want to improve their control and manage their breath in a variety of settings, including sexual relations.

Box breathing is a valuable breathing technique for individuals seeking to regulate their breath, enhance control, and manage stress, especially in the context of sexual encounters. Its structured and balanced nature makes it a practical tool that can be easily integrated into pre-sexual rituals or used as a grounding technique during intimate moments. Regular practice and adaptation to individual preferences contribute to maximizing the benefits of this breathing technique.

Key components of Box Breathing include:

1. Equal Duration Phases: Individuals start by inhaling slowly and deeply through the nose, typically for a count of four. After the inhalation, there is a pause or hold of the breath, maintaining the same count (e.g., four counts). Exhalation follows, with individuals exhaling slowly and completely through the mouth or nose for the same count (e.g., four counts).

The cycle concludes with another breath-holding phase, maintaining the same count as before.

2. Structured and Controlled Breathing: By emphasizing a structured and controlled rhythm, box breathing enables people to create a pattern of intentional and purposeful breathing. An even breathing cycle is facilitated by the identical length of each phase. The neurological system may feel more at ease as a result of this equilibrium.

3. Box breathing is very helpful for controlling breathing during intercourse. This method's deliberate and balanced approach can offset fast or erratic breathing linked to elevated arousal. Box breathing encourages controlled and rhythmic breathing, which can help improve control over physiological reactions, such as arousal levels.

4. Stress and Anxiety Management: By triggering the parasympathetic nervous system, box breathing encourages a state of relaxation. This may help with stress and anxiety management, which is relevant when it comes to sexual engagement. Box breathing is a grounded method that helps people stay in the present moment and focused because of its regulated form.

5. People can use box breathing in their pre-sexual rituals. They can use it as a calming technique to center themselves before having intimate moments. Box breathing can be made more effective with frequent practice, just like other breathing techniques. Maintaining consistency helps people get more comfortable with the technique, which makes it easier to use when things get stressful.

Advantages of Controlled Box Breathing:

Box breathing's regulated breathing pattern can help control excitement levels and stop rapid or erratic breathing.

Inducing a relaxation response through box breathing lowers stress levels and makes the environment cozier.

Box breathing's disciplined rhythm helps improve concentration and focus, fostering a more aware and in-the-moment attitude.

Box breathing is a useful and accessible technique that people can covertly employ in a variety of settings, including private ones.

Visualization and Mental Conditioning

1. Positive Outcome Visualization:

Mental conditioning and visualization entail the purposeful construction of scenarios and mental images to favorably affect attitudes, feelings, and actions. Using positive result visualization in the breathing for control context is an effective method. A useful part of mental conditioning is positive result imagery, which gives people a way to deal with their worry and boost their self-esteem when it comes to premature ejaculation. This method becomes a comprehensive strategy for promoting a positive outlook, lowering fear, and improving general control during intimate moments when combined with breathing techniques. To get the most out of mental training and visualization, regular practice is essential.

Important Elements:

1. Positive Outcome Visualization: People consciously conjure up ideas in their minds of fulfilling and successful sex. To do this, picture yourself having extended sexual activity without ejaculating too soon. The goal is to create a good mental association with sex by focusing on imagining success and satisfaction. This can help

dispel nervous or negative ideas about ejaculating too soon.

2. Reframing Worrying Thoughts: One way to deal with performance anxiety is through visualization. People can reframe anxious thoughts and cultivate a more optimistic mindset by imagining good possibilities. Imagining positive outcomes helps people become more confident in their capacity to manage and enjoy sexual encounters. This psychological programming encourages an assertive and proactive stance.

3. Application to Premature Ejaculation: Performance anxiety is frequently linked to premature ejaculation. Visualization provides a method for lowering this anxiety through mental rehearsal of favorable outcomes.
favorable associations are formed with sexual experiences when favorable results are envisioned. This psychological training may help break the pattern of worry and early ejaculation.

4. Integration with Breathing Techniques: Breathing techniques and visualization can coexist together. For example, people can enhance the total influence on mental and physiological states by practicing controlled breathing while visualizing

positive outcomes. When breathing exercises and visualization are combined, it improves relaxation and leads to a more happy and in control emotional state during sexual activity.

Advantages of Visualizing Positive Outcomes

Anxiety Reduction: By giving people a mental tool to handle performance-related stress, visualization can reduce anxiety related to premature ejaculation.

Self-assurance: People can develop self-assurance in their capacity to regulate and relish sexual encounters by regularly imagining favorable results.

Positive outcome imagery plays a role in mental conditioning by establishing a favorable link with sexual encounters and encouraging proactivity.

Integration with Breathing: Visualization improves control and relaxation when paired with breathing techniques, providing a comprehensive method of treating early ejaculation.

2. Mental Conditioning Scripts:
Creating structured mental narratives with adaptive reactions to possible obstacles and positive affirmations is known as mental conditioning

scripting. These scripts are a proactive tool for mental conditioning that assist people in developing resilience and confidence, particularly when it comes to performance-related issues like early ejaculation.

Scripts for mental conditioning are a proactive means for people to improve their mental readiness, especially when it comes to early ejaculation. These scripts help with anxiety reduction, resilience development, and confidence building by including adaptive reactions and positive affirmations. To fully reap the benefits of mental conditioning scripts, practice must be done on a regular and consistent basis.

Important Elements:

1. Positive Affirmations: Positive affirmations that bolster self-assurance and confidence are a part of mental scripts. These affirmations help cultivate a more optimistic outlook by dispelling unfavorable ideas. The goal of affirmations is to increase self-confidence in one's capacity for both control and enjoyment of sex. The mental conditioning for improved performance is supported by this positive reinforcement.

2. Adaptive Reactions to Difficulties: Scripts tackle any difficulties or worries about ejaculating too soon. This anticipatory quality enables people to mentally get ready for a range of situations. Adaptive reactions to difficulties are part of the mental conditioning scripts. These reactions could entail breathing exercises, changing the way one is thinking, or shifting attention to the good parts of the encounter.

3. Repetition and Consistency: Regular practice is necessary for mental conditioning scripts to be successful. People regularly reinforce adaptive reactions and positive affirmations by repeating these scripts.
Scripts are incorporated into everyday activities and grow to be a second nature to mental preparation. The script's effect on performance and mindset is enhanced by this regular practice.

Advantages of Scripts for Mental Conditioning:

Scripts with positive affirmations help develop self-efficacy and confidence, both of which are necessary for handling performance-related issues.

Adaptive reactions in scripts offer proactive approaches to overcome obstacles, which aid in the development of resilience in people.

Anxiety is lessened and a sense of preparedness for impending pressures is created by anticipating difficulties and having prepared answers in scripts. Mental conditioning scripts that are often repeated promote constructive attitudes and behaviors, which helps create long-lasting mental shifts.

3. Cue-Controlled Relaxation:

Creating certain signals, such a touch or phrase, that serve as triggers for a relaxation response is known as cue-controlled relaxation. This method, which is a component of mental conditioning, allows people to regulate their arousal levels during sexual engagement by acting as an anchor for relaxation.

A specific method within mental conditioning called cue-controlled relaxation gives people a useful tool for anchoring relaxation during sexual activity. A person's capacity to regulate arousal and prevent premature ejaculation can be improved by incorporating certain cues into intimate times and linking them with a relaxed mood. This strategy is particularly effective when used in conjunction with regular practice and customized cue selection.

Important Elements:

1. Creating Relaxation signals: People select particular signals that they associate with relaxation and calmness, such as a soft touch, a specific word, or a particular breathing pattern. A specific list of cues is chosen depending on what the client finds relaxing and connects with them.

2. Association with Relaxation: Through deliberate pairing, the selected cues are connected to relaxation. The cue could be presented, for instance, when one is calm or in tandem with relaxing methods. By teaching the mind to respond to these signals with a soothing impact, repetition strengthens the association between the cues and a relaxed state.

3. Application during Sexual Activity: During sexual interactions, the recognized cues are included. They act as cues to the mind and body to start a relaxation response when they are introduced. People can keep control over their arousal levels and avoid the escalation of stress or anxiety that

comes with premature ejaculation by practicing cue-controlled relaxation.

Advantages of Cue-Controlled Relaxation

Immediate Relaxation reaction: Cues cause people to experience an instantaneous relaxation reaction, which enables them to instantly control stress and anxiety during private moments.

Improved Control: Using certain cues offers a concrete way to keep a handle on arousal levels, which helps to improve total ejaculatory control.

Personalization and Adaptability: Cue-controlled relaxation is incredibly flexible, enabling users to select cues that speak to them directly, which increases the method's efficacy.

Cues can be smoothly incorporated into pre-sexual rituals once they are established, becoming an organic and regular part of the person's day.

4. Desensitization via Visualization:
This technique entails exposing them to sexual situations progressively through mental images. By gradually desensitizing people to anxiety-inducing conditions associated with sexual performance, this

methodical technique seeks to increase ejaculatory control and lessen performance-related stress. A calculated approach to lowering performance-related stress and enhancing ejaculatory control is desensitization by visualization.

Using a controlled mental environment, people are gradually exposed to many sexual scenarios, which fosters familiarity, confidence, and resilience. As part of a comprehensive strategy to manage premature ejaculation, regular and methodical practice improves the efficiency of desensitization through visualization.

It's key elements includes:

1. Gradual Exposure: Visualization entails exposing oneself to various sexual scenarios one at a time, beginning with less stressful ones and working your way up to more difficult ones. Because the procedure is methodical, people can progressively adjust to varying degrees of intensity in the events they've envisioned.

2. Anxiety Reduction: By exposing people to a variety of sexual situations, visualization helps them become less anxious about the novelty and

unpredictability that might cause anxiety.Desensitization focuses on particular apprehensions about sexual performance, including the dread of ejaculating too soon, and enables people to face and deal with these worries in a safe mental space.

3. Improving Ejaculatory Control: By using mental training scripts or focused breathing exercises, people can improve their ejaculatory control during visualization. Building Good Connections:* Gradual exposure combined with effective visualization produces

4. Pleasant Associations: Successful visualization and gradual exposure foster pleasant associations with sexual situations, which encourage a more assured and restrained approach to private times.

Advantages of Visualization-Based Desensitization:

1. Decreased Performance-Related Stress: By acquainting people with various situations, visualization aids in the reduction of anxiety and stress related to sexual performance.

2. Enhanced Confidence: The methodical desensitization process helps people feel more

confident about their capacity to manage different parts of sexual interactions.

3. Enhanced Control Methodologies: Visualization offers a safe space to hone control methods before implementing them in practical settings.

4. Flexibility to Meet Individual Needs: The procedure can be tailored to meet the needs of each person, taking into account their comfort levels and particular concerns.

Assurance-based methods include mental training approaches, breathing exercises, and mindfulness. By incorporating these methods into a holistic strategy for controlling premature ejaculation, people can be better equipped to develop positive thinking, improve control over their body's reactions, and have more fulfilling sex. Persistent application and customized modification of these methods can lead to sustained enhancements in ejaculatory regulation and general sexual health.

Chapter Four: Communication and Partner Involvement

Importance of Open Communication

The first step in treating premature ejaculation is open conversation. It offers a forum for people to share their ideas, worries, and emotions regarding their encounters. One cannot stress the value of candid communication while dealing with early ejaculation. In the end, it contributes to a healthier and more meaningful sexual relationship between partners by serving as the foundation for mutual understanding, cooperative problem-solving, and the creation of emotional safety.

Aspects of open communication:

1. Shared Understanding: When partners communicate openly, a shared understanding is fostered. Talking freely about premature ejaculation enables both parties to express their feelings, worries, and ideas. Because of this transparency, both parties can better understand one another's expectations and points of view on the matter.

2. The second step is normalizing the discourse about sexual health for partners to talk openly about premature ejaculation. Speaking out about the situation helps both parties deal with it more compassionately and understandingly and lessens stigma.

3. Trigger Identification: People are able to pinpoint probable causes or aggravating circumstances for early ejaculation by being candid with each other. Building focused strategies and solutions to successfully address the problem requires an understanding of the underlying reasons.

4. Collaborative Issue-Solving: Cooperative issue-solving is made possible by candid communication. Whether the solutions entail making lifestyle adjustments, undergoing psychiatric counseling, or consulting a professional, partners can collaborate to investigate alternate options. The relationship between partners is reinforced by this cooperative strategy.

5. Deeper Emotional Connection: Discussing ideas and emotions around early ejaculation leads to a more profound emotional bond. The openness with which such personal matters are discussed fosters a sense of trust and intimacy between spouses.

6. Clarification of Expectations: Open communication enables partners to discuss what they expect from their sex. A more fulfilling sexual relationship results from both parties being aware of each other's needs, preferences, and worries. This helps control expectations.

7. Reduction of Performance Anxiety: Premature ejaculation can be openly discussed to aid with performance anxiety. Open communication between partners about their experiences reduces the pressure to perform sexually and creates a supportive environment for both parties.

8. Establishing Emotional Safety: Emotional safety is established through fostering an environment of candid dialogue. People feel comfortable talking about their worries without worrying about being judged, which creates a safe space for discussing and handling early ejaculation.

9. Mutual Support is Facilitated: Mutual support is facilitated by open communication. Partners can help navigate the difficulties presented by premature ejaculation by offering emotional support, empathy, and encouragement. This fosters a sense of community.

10. Encouragement to Seek Help: Talking about early ejaculation can make people realize how helpful it is to get expert assistance. A complete approach to addressing the issue is promoted by open communication, which encourages individuals to consider consulting healthcare doctors or sexual health experts.

2. Cutting Down on Stigma:

One of the most important ways to cut down on stigma and create a welcoming and compassionate atmosphere is to have candid conversations about early ejaculation. One essential component of fostering a caring and understanding atmosphere is lowering the stigma associated with early ejaculation. With an end goal of enhancing general well-being and relationship satisfaction, candid conversations question social conventions, advance education, and give people the confidence to ask for assistance.

Key points about reducing stigma are as follows:

1. The process of normalizing premature ejaculation as a common occurrence is aided by candid conversations. People experience less feelings of guilt and loneliness when they talk about and acknowledge it as a normal part of sexual wellness.

2. Challenging Social Taboos: Social taboos and misunderstandings have frequently surrounded premature ejaculation. By challenging these taboos, candid discussions help to advance a more realistic and knowledgeable perspective of sexual health.

3. Promoting Empathy: Empathy is increased through open communication. Partners learn more about each other's feelings, struggles, and experiences when they talk about premature ejaculation. This empathy fosters a dynamic that is more sympathetic and encouraging.

4. Encouraging Education: Honest conversations offer a chance for education. Couples can debunk myths and false information by learning about the several reasons that lead to premature ejaculation. Because it spreads accurate facts, education is essential in lowering stigma.

5. Empowering People: Having an honest conversation regarding early ejaculation gives people the power to take charge of their sexual well-being. It promotes proactively looking for answers, whether by alterations to one's way of life, therapeutic interventions, or expert advice.

6. Destigmatizing Help Seeking: Talking honestly about early ejaculation helps to de-stigmatize the act of seeking assistance. It conveys the idea that taking care of one's sexual health is a natural and responsible part of overall wellbeing, empowering people to seek competent advice without feeling judged.

7. Establishing a Safe Space: Honest discussions foster a place where people can talk about their experiences without worrying about being judged. Collaboratively treating and managing premature ejaculation requires this safe environment.

8. Developing Resilience: One way to develop resilience is to lessen stigma. People are more capable of overcoming the difficulties presented by early ejaculation when they feel heard and supported, which encourages an optimistic and proactive outlook.

9. Improving Relationship Dynamics: Relationship dynamics are strengthened when candid conversations regarding early ejaculation are had. Relationships that are healthier, closer, and more trustworthy are those in which partners discuss sexual health in an honest and encouraging manner.

10. Cultural Shift in Perspectives: One factor influencing this shift in viewpoint is ongoing, honest discussion regarding early ejaculation. This change may eventually result in a more accepting and compassionate society perspective on sexual health.

3. Finding Solutions:

Partners can work together to find viable answers to the problem of early ejaculation by keeping lines of communication open. This procedure entails experimenting with several methods, such as modifying one's lifestyle, using psychological techniques, and consulting a specialist. When coming up with strategies together to deal with premature ejaculation, open communication is essential. People can collaborate to identify tactics that suit their demands and enhance a more fulfilling sexual connection by trying out different methods and incorporating both parties in the process.

The following are important considerations while identifying solutions:

1. Holistic Exploration: When partners communicate openly, they can approach problem-solving from a holistic perspective. They

can investigate several variables that could lead to early ejaculation, taking into account both physiological and psychological elements.

2. Lifestyle Modifications: Couples can talk about and put into practice lifestyle modifications that could help prevent early ejaculation. This may entail modifying one's food, exercise regimen, and sleeping schedule in an effort to enhance general health and wellbeing.

3. Psychological Strategies: Open communication fosters discussions about psychological strategies. Couples might investigate methods like mental training, mindfulness, and relaxation exercises to treat psychological issues causing early ejaculation.

4. Behavioral Interventions: Considering behavioral interventions is made possible by candid communication. Couples can work together to perform exercises that are designed to enhance ejaculatory control; these exercises may include methods that have been prescribed by therapists or medical professionals.

5. Professional Guidance: When partners discuss early ejaculation candidly, it encourages them to think about getting professional advice. This could

entail speaking with medical professionals, specialists in sexual health, or therapists who can offer specific guidance and treatments.

6. Examining Sexual practices: Partners are free to explore and talk about sexual practices that could improve satisfaction and control. Trying out various strategies, communication philosophies, and degrees of closeness might help identify solutions that benefit both parties.

7. Tracking Progress: Finding answers necessitates a dedication to tracking advancement. Partners can evaluate the success of tactics being implemented, make necessary adjustments, and recognize progress by keeping in constant communication.

8. Flexibility and adaptability: When finding answers, open communication promotes flexibility and adaptability. It could be necessary for partners to experiment with various tactics, and being flexible enough to adjust to evolving situations enhances the effectiveness of all the tactics used.

9. Emphasis on Shared accountability: Shared accountability is emphasized during the solution-finding process. The proactive involvement of both partners in devising and

executing methods promotes a shared
understanding of how to tackle the obstacles caused
by early ejaculation.

10. Fostering Emotional Bond: When partners work
together to find solutions, their emotional bond is
strengthened. The mutual dedication to devising
successful tactics strengthens the connection
overall and fosters a positive dynamic.

4. Emotional Connection:

Fostering an open line of communication is
essential to maintaining an emotional bond
between spouses. Sharing vulnerabilities,
encouraging closeness, and fortifying the
relationship as a whole are all part of this process.
The foundation of a strong and happy relationship
is the emotional bond that is created by honest
communication. Partners build a solid basis for
closeness, resiliency, and long-term enjoyment in
their relationship by being vulnerable with one
another, appreciating one another's viewpoints, and
showing empathy and support for one another.

It's significance include:

1. Vulnerability and Authenticity: Partners who communicate openly are more inclined to be honest and open about their emotions and experiences. People connect more deeply when they are able to be authentic without worrying about being judged.

2. Trust-Building: Open communication between partners fosters trust. People build trust when they feel comfortable sharing their ideas and feelings, which makes a relationship feel more stable and secure.

3. Mutual Understanding: Understanding between people is facilitated by open communication. Open communication between partners helps them understand one another better by gaining insights into one another's experiences, especially those pertaining to premature ejaculation. This fosters empathy and a deeper understanding of one another.

4. Empathy and Support: Sharing one's weaknesses and worries encourages empathy and support. Open communication between partners regarding problems like early ejaculation increases the

likelihood that they will console, support, and understand one another.

5. Shared Experiences: Partners can traverse shared experiences by having an open discussion. Talking about private issues like early ejaculation establishes a shared path and promotes a sense of unity and connection when overcoming obstacles as a group.

6. Enhanced Intimacy: Enhanced intimacy is influenced by emotional connection. A partner's degree of intimacy is positively impacted by their emotional connection, which fosters a deeper and more meaningful bond in both routine and intimate interactions.

7. Building Relationship Resilience: Relationship resilience is bolstered by a solid emotional bond. Open communication and the development of strong emotional links between partners make it easier for them to overcome obstacles and overcome problems, especially those pertaining to their sexual health.

8. Promoting Emotional Expression: Emotional expression is promoted by open conversation. Free communication between partners about their

pleasures, worries, and desires creates a supportive atmosphere where feelings are recognized and respected.

9. Conflict settlement: A key component of conflict settlement is emotional ties. Emotionally close partners are more inclined to approach disagreements with empathy and a desire to work together to create win-win solutions.

10. Long-Term Satisfaction: Long-term relationship satisfaction is linked to a strong emotional bond. Open communication helps partners build strong emotional ties, and these couples typically feel more fulfilled and pleased in their relationships.

Involving the Partner in the Process

In order to treat premature ejaculation and turn it from a personal problem into a shared experience, partner engagement is essential. Including the partner in the process of dealing with early ejaculation is a comprehensive strategy that turns the difficulty into a joint adventure. It creates a sense of shared accountability, strengthens understanding between the parties, motivates engagement, nurtures compassion and support, improves communication, increases closeness, and unites the two parties toward shared objectives.

This cooperative endeavor not only resolves the particular problem but also improves the dynamics of the relationships in general.

The important factors include:

1. Shared Responsibility: Involving partners highlights that ejaculating too soon is a shared concern that calls for cooperation. Recognizing this shared accountability encourages cooperation and unity as a team to overcome the obstacle. The emphasis is shifted from individual struggle to group problem-solving through this collaborative approach.

2. Comprehending Partner Needs: Involving a partner requires a deeper comprehension of their needs and preferences. Open communication allows partners to discuss and clarify expectations, which lays the groundwork for coming up with solutions that work for both of them. This shared understanding creates a framework for handling premature ejaculation while taking both partners' needs and preferences into account.

3. Taking Part in Solutions: One of the most important aspects of partner involvement is taking an active part in solutions. Partners take an active

role in the process by participating in activities, going to treatment sessions, or encouraging lifestyle adjustments. This collaborative effort strengthens commitment and increases the efficacy of the selected strategies. It furthers the notion that both partners are essential in preventing early ejaculation, encouraging cooperation and shared responsibility for the result.

4. Empathy and Support: Involving a partner helps to develop empathy and support. Being aware of how early ejaculation affects the partner's mental health enables one to react with greater compassion. By accepting and supporting one another's experiences, partners can offer each other emotional support. This empathy fosters a caring atmosphere where people feel heard and understood contributing to a positive and nurturing dynamic.

5. Improved Communication: Involving the spouse improves communication. It is recommended that partners have an honest conversation about their thoughts, feelings, and experiences about early ejaculation. By fostering a climate of openness and trust, this enhanced communication not only helps people understand one another better but also improves the relationship as a whole.

6. Developing Intimacy: Intimacy can be developed through partner interaction. The shared experiences that arise from tackling problems together and actively contributing to solutions strengthen the emotional and physical bond between spouses. Overcoming challenges together deepens the relationship and creates a sense of connection that transcends the particular problem of early ejaculation.

7. Shared Objectives and Advancement: When a partner participates, both parties work toward common objectives. Establishing agreed goals and keeping track of advancements fosters a sense of accomplishment and mutual success. Celebrating victories strengthens the bond between partners by reiterating the notion that overcoming early ejaculation is a shared achievement.

Building a Supportive Environment

It's essential to have a supportive environment for people who experience premature ejaculation. This entails establishing emotional security, supporting others in asking for assistance, giving encouragement, adjusting as a team, and preserving closeness. In order to create a supportive environment, it is important to put emotional safety first, encourage getting professional treatment when needed, give positive reinforcement, adjust as a team, and keep closeness. This all-encompassing strategy buil

ds a foundation for people to deal with early ejaculation together, encouraging mutual growth, understanding, and resilience in the relationship.

Elements of building a supportive environment include:

1. Emotional Safety: A welcoming atmosphere places a high value on candid communication, enabling people to share their worries, anxieties, and experiences without worrying about being judged. A higher level of connection between spouses is fostered by this emotional safety, which provides an environment where vulnerability is embraced. In a nurturing environment, partners actively hear and affirm each other's emotions. It is easier to foster a nonjudgmental environment where people feel heard and supported when they are aware of the emotional effects of premature ejaculation.

2. Encouraging Seeking Help: In a nurturing setting, getting professional assistance is no longer

stigmatized. The possible advantages of speaking with therapists, medical professionals, or specialists in sexual health can be freely discussed among partners. The perception that asking for help is a proactive and wise decision is reinforced by supporting this action. A sense of cooperation and shared responsibility is strengthened when both parties are involved in the decision-making process, whether it is about treatment, medical interventions, or lifestyle modifications.

3. Positive Reinforcement: In a supportive setting, providing positive reinforcement is crucial. Honoring successes, no matter how minor, makes the environment happier. By fostering a sense of accomplishment and group success, acknowledging progress strengthens resilience and motivation. Prioritizing efforts over results creates a positive and encouraging environment. Acknowledging the perseverance and commitment to dealing with early ejaculation strengthens team dynamics and promotes continued cooperation.

4. Adapting Together: Adaptability is welcomed in a supportive setting. Each pair should be willing to try out various tactics and work collaboratively to adjust their strategies as needed. Continuous progress and an openness to trying out novel ideas

are made possible by flexibility. Overcoming obstacles as a group fosters resilience and problem-solving skills. Partners actively participate in problem solving in a supportive environment, fostering a collaborative style that deepens their relationship.

5. Maintaining Intimacy: Upholding intimacy is important, even in the face of difficulties brought on by early ejaculation. To maintain a happy and meaningful relationship, partners can experiment with different types of intimacy, concentrating on emotional connection, shared experiences, and non-sexual bonding.
It's important to discuss intimacy wants and desires in an open manner. In order to create a supportive atmosphere that goes beyond the particular problem of early ejaculation, partners can talk about their preferences, worries, and methods to improve their emotional and physical connection.

When it comes to treating premature ejaculation, communication and partner involvement are essential. Transparency in communication lays the groundwork for understanding, and involving the partner turns the problem into a cooperative endeavor. Creating a welcoming atmosphere fosters empathy, flexibility, and a shared dedication to

coming up with workable solutions. When
combined, these components offer a comprehensive
strategy for handling early ejaculation in the
framework of a compassionate and understanding
relationship.

Chapter Five: Natural Remedies and Supplements for Premature Ejaculation

Certain natural therapies and supplements can sometimes be used to treat premature ejaculation. The following is a list of necessary nutrients, natural medicines, and supplements that support sexual health and function:

Medicinal Herbs for Sexual Wellness

1. Tribulus Terrestris

Due to its possible advantages for sexual health, Tribulus Terrestris is a plant that has been utilized traditionally in a number of traditional medical systems. Its capacity to raise testosterone levels is frequently cited as the reason for its significance in sexual health. It is thought that Tribulus Terrestris increases luteinizing hormone (LH) production, which instructs the testes to create more testosterone. Improved sexual function and an enhanced libido are linked to higher testosterone levels.

Its potential benefits include:

1. Increased Libido: Tribulus Terrestris is frequently recommended as having aphrodisiac qualities that may increase arousal or libido.

2. Enhanced Testosterone Levels: Tribulus terrestris may enhance testosterone levels, which are essential for general sexual function, by altering the production of LH.

3. Although certain research indicates possible advantages, there is inconclusive data on Tribulus Terrestris' efficacy in promoting sexual health. Individual reactions might differ, and additional study is required to conclusively determine its effectiveness.

2. Ashwagandha

Traditionally used in medicine, ashwagandha, also called Withania somnifera, is an adaptogenic herb. Its function is linked to lowering stress and promoting general wellbeing, both of which can benefit sexual health. The key to ashwagandha's ability to reduce stress is its adaptogenic qualities. Ashwagandha is thought to modify the body's stress response, especially by lowering cortisol levels. Adaptogens are drugs that assist the body in adapting to stresses.

Traditional medicine favors ashwagandha because of its adaptogenic properties and capacity to reduce stress. Ashwagandha has the ability to enhance overall well-being by regulating the body's stress response, which could have positive effects on other facets of health, including sexual well-being. As with any supplement, specific precautions and expert advice are necessary for safe and effective use.

Potential benefits:
1. Regulation of Cortisol: When under stress, the hormone cortisol is released. Ashwagandha may provide a healthy stress response by assisting in the regulation of cortisol levels.

2. Alleviation of Anxiety: Ashwagandha is thought to have anxiolytic (anxiety-reducing) properties by influencing neurotransmitters and the nervous system. This may help to lessen anxiety related to sexual performance.

3. Improved Overall Well-Being:.Overall well-being may be enhanced by ashwagandha's stress-relieving properties. Stress management is essential for preserving emotional and mental balance, which tangentially supports many facets of health, including sexual wellness.

4. Stress reduction with ashwagandha may lead to a happier and more optimistic outlook, which are associated with general well-being.

5. As an adaptogen, ashwagandha may assist in regulating energy levels, avoiding extreme exhaustion or burnout that may interfere with regular activities, such as engaging in sexual engagement.

3. Maca Root
Known by its scientific name, Lepidium meyenii, maca is a root vegetable that is indigenous to Peru. It has become more well-known due to its possible advantages for sexual health, and it is frequently linked to increased libido and better sexual performance.

Maca root is known for its ability to balance hormones, increase libido, and boost endurance and stamina. Although its aphrodisiac properties have long been known, individual reactions may differ. For best effects, as with any herbal supplement, it's important to approach Maca from a balanced standpoint, taking into account individual factors, dose, and expert advice.

Its roles include:
1. Increasing Libido: Maca is said to possess adaptogenic qualities, which means it could assist the body in adjusting to stress and balancing different systems, such as the endocrine system. It

is believed that this equilibrium has a role in heightened libido or sexual desire.

Maca is known to have aphrodisiac properties, meaning it may heighten arousal or desire for sex.

2. Addressing Hormonal Balance: It is believed that Maca interacts with the endocrine system to affect hormonal balance. This covers possible impacts on hormones like testosterone, progesterone, and estrogen. Maca may help maintain hormonal balance, which is essential for overall reproductive health, by regulating the endocrine system.

3. Increasing Stamina and Endurance: Maca's supporters contend that it may have a favorable impact on energy levels and endurance, which would help with stamina-related problems. Some people think that maca increases energy, which could help with endurance during physical activities like sex. Maca's adaptogenic qualities might help people have greater endurance, which would enable them to exert themselves physically for longer periods of time.

5. Ginseng

There is a long-standing belief that ginseng, especially Panax ginseng, might enhance sexual performance. Its action is linked to increasing the synthesis of nitric oxide, which may have a beneficial effect on blood flow and maybe assist erectile function. It has long been known to have the ability to improve blood flow and nitric oxide production, which can both improve sexual performance. Although there might be advantages for sexual health, safe and efficient use requires individual considerations, appropriate dosages, and professional advice.

1. It is thought that ginseng helps the body produce more nitric oxide. A signaling molecule called nitric oxide aids in blood vessel dilatation and enhances blood flow. Ginseng may help improve vasodilation and improve blood circulation throughout the body, including the genital area, by raising nitric oxide levels.

2. Promotion of Better Blood Flow: Ginseng is linked to enhanced blood flow, which may have advantageous effects on erectile function. Enough blood flow to the penis is necessary to initiate and sustain an erection. Ginseng may improve erectile function by increasing blood flow, which may help with erectile dysfunction-related problems.

3. General Vitality: Since ginseng is frequently considered an adaptogen, it may aid the body in adjusting to stress. Ginseng may have an indirect effect on sexual health by fostering a general sense of vitality and well-being. The adaptogenic qualities of ginseng may help with vigor and energy levels, which may help with exhaustion or low energy that may impair sexual performance.

There are several varieties of ginseng, but Panax ginseng is the kind that has been researched the most for possible health advantages. Selecting a trustworthy source for ginseng supplements is very essential.

5. Horny Goat Weed (Epimedium)

Scientifically termed Epimedium, Horny Goat Weed may have advantages for the health of the sex. Its function is frequently linked to enhancing blood flow to the genital area, which can lead to better sexual performance and erectile function. It is thought that horny goat weed improves vaginal blood flow, which benefits sexual wellness.

Although it has been used historically as an aphrodisiac and to improve erotic performance, safe and efficient use requires individual considerations, appropriate dosages, and professional direction.

1. Better Blood Flow: It is believed that chemicals in horny goat weed may encourage vasodilation, which is the process of widening blood vessels. An increase in blood flow to the vaginal area may result from this process. Improved blood flow is one way that Horny Goat Weed may help with erectile dysfunction. For the purpose of getting and keeping an erection during sexual activity, this is essential.

2. Support for Sexual Performance: Horny Goat Weed's enhanced blood flow may have a favorable effect on a person's ability to perform sexually overall. Several facets of sexual health depend on adequate blood flow. Enhanced libido, a crucial element of whole sexual performance, can be attributed to elevated blood flow. Horny Goat Weed might help people stay strong by promoting blood circulation during sexual activity, potentially addressing concerns related to premature fatigue.

3. Horny Goat Weed has been traditionally regarded as an aphrodisiac, with historical use in traditional medicine systems for its potential to boost sexual desire.

The herb's reputation as an aphrodisiac suggests that it may have properties that stimulate or enhance sexual desire.

6. Ginkgo Biloba

This herb is well-known for improving blood circulation and is frequently linked to improving vascular health in general. Ginkgo Biloba's claimed increase in blood flow may have effects on erectile dysfunction and general sexual wellness.
The potential benefits of Ginkgo Biloba for vascular health and enhanced blood circulation may extend to improved erectile performance and overall sexual health. As with any supplement, safe and efficient use depends on individual factors, appropriate dosages, and expert advice.

1. Better Blood Circulation: It is thought that ginkgo biloba has vasodilatory properties, which expand blood vessels and improve blood flow. Enhancing circulation has multiple health benefits, including those associated with sexual wellness. Ginkgo Biloba may help with erectile dysfunction by improving blood flow. To achieve and maintain an erection, enough blood circulation is essential.

2. Support for Vascular Health: Ginkgo Biloba's beneficial effects on blood vessels also extend to the support of vascular health. The body needs healthy blood vessels to carry nutrients and oxygen throughout it. Arousal, responsiveness, and contentment are just a few of the characteristics of sexual health that can benefit from improved vascular health.

3. Cognitive Enhancement: Ginkgo Biloba has been shown to have potential cognitive-enhancing benefits, despite having no direct connection to sexual health. A pleasurable sexual encounter may be indirectly influenced by improved cognitive performance. The effects of Ginkgo Biloba on cognitive function may enhance mental health in general and may have an impact on sexual health.

It's important to take supplements medications as directed. Overindulgence may not always result in more benefits and may even have negative repercussions. Selecting a reliable source for supplements is essential to guaranteeing the product's effectiveness and purity.

Essential Nutrients and their Role

1. Zinc
Zinc is a necessary mineral that is important for several physiological functions, with hormone balancing and general reproductive health being two of these functions.
The synthesis of testosterone and the fact that zinc is found in reproductive organs highlight zinc's significance for preserving hormonal balance and promoting general reproductive health. Zinc requirements for optimal sexual and reproductive health can be met in part by eating a well-balanced diet and, if necessary, taking the right supplements.

1. Production of Testosterone: A crucial male sex hormone, testosterone, is synthesized and regulated in part by zinc. A number of components of reproductive health, such as sperm production and general sexual function, depend heavily on testosterone. Sufficient zinc levels support the preservation of hormonal equilibrium, which guarantees the best possible testosterone production for healthy reproductive processes.
The development and maturation of sperm cells depend on zinc. Enough zinc promotes the growth of healthy sperm, which is essential for reproduction.

2. Reproductive Health: The testes and prostate, two male reproductive organs, have substantial levels of zinc. Its significance in sustaining the composition and operation of these organs is highlighted by their dispersion. The prostate gland benefits from zinc for both health and optimal operation. Prostate health maintenance is important for overall reproductive health.

Dietary Sources:
Meat, dairy products, nuts, and seeds are just a few of the foods that contain zinc. Meeting zinc needs involves eating a balanced diet that include these sources. Supplementation may be taken into consideration when there is a possible inadequacy in food intake or when there is a particular worry over zinc levels. However, prior to beginning any supplementation, it is imperative that you speak with a healthcare provider.

The amount of zinc that is advised to be consumed daily varies depending on age, sex, and health. Optimizing zinc benefits requires attending to individual needs.

2. Vitamin D

An essential fat-soluble vitamin, vitamin D has a significant effect on many aspects of health, including testosterone levels and possible effects on reproductive health. The importance of vitamin D for reproductive health is highlighted by its correlation with testosterone levels as well as its roles in immune system and bone health. Getting enough vitamin D via sunshine, eating a healthy diet, or taking supplements can help with reproductive health and general well-being.

1. Testosterone Levels: Cells that generate testosterone have vitamin D receptors. Sufficient quantities of vitamin D are believed to maintain these cells' regular functions, which impact the synthesis and control of testosterone. Making sure you have enough vitamin D may help you keep your testosterone levels at their ideal levels, which supports hormonal balance and reproductive health.

2. Bone Health and Calcium Absorption: In the intestines, calcium absorption is greatly aided by vitamin D. This is necessary to preserve the integrity of the entire skeleton and the health of the bones. Vitamin D supports appropriate bone density maintenance by encouraging the absorption

of calcium. This is crucial for general health and could have a knock-on effect on areas of sexual health.

3. Immune System Function: The immune system is supported by vitamin D, which is well-known. Having a strong immune system is essential for general health and wellness. Vitamin D enhances immunity, which benefits general health. A healthy body is better able to sustain its ideal level of reproduction.

Sun Exposure: When exposed to sunlight, the body creates vitamin D. Vitamin D synthesis can be boosted by exposure to sunlight and outdoor activities.

Dietary Sources:
Certain foods, such as fatty fish, fortified dairy products, and some mushrooms, contain vitamin D. Consuming these sources of vitamin D aids in meeting daily needs. Vitamin D supplementation may be taken into consideration in cases where exposure to sunlight and dietary consumption may not be sufficient. As with any supplement, it's best to speak with a healthcare provider.

The amount of vitamin D that each person needs varies. Age, skin tone, region, and state of health are some of the variables that affect the body's capacity to make and absorb vitamin D.

3. Omega-3 Fatty Acids

Polyunsaturated fats, such as omega-3 fatty acids, are essential for maintaining cardiovascular health, and studies on this area of health may also enhance sexual function. The importance of omega-3 fatty acids for sexual performance is highlighted by their ability to lower inflammation, promote cardiovascular health, and possibly even affect mood. Reproductive health and general well-being can be enhanced by include foods high in omega-3s in the diet or by thinking about taking supplements while eating a balanced diet.

1. Cardiovascular Health: By lowering inflammation, enhancing blood vessel function, and promoting heart health, omega-3 fatty acids help to maintain cardiovascular health. For the body's blood to flow properly throughout, healthy blood vessels are necessary. Omega-3 fatty acids may have a beneficial effect on blood flow to the vaginal area by supporting normal blood vessel function. For an erection to occur, enough blood circulation is essential. Numerous cardiovascular problems are

linked to inflammation. The anti-inflammatory qualities of omega-3s may support heart health in general, which may have an indirect effect on sexual function.

2. Brain Health and Mood: Essential elements of brain cell membranes are omega-3 fatty acids. They may have an impact on mood and mental health because they are involved in neurotransmitter activity. The benefits of omega-3 fatty acids for brain function may extend to mood and mental wellness. Sexual health and psychological aspects are interwoven. Omega-3 fatty acids might have a calming effect on stress, which could influence things like performance anxiety, which can affect a person's ability to mate.

Dietary Sources:
Walnuts, flaxseeds, chia seeds, and fatty fish (such salmon and mackerel) are good sources of omega-3 fatty acids. Consuming these foods increases consumption of omega-3 fatty acids.
When dietary consumption appears to be inadequate, omega-3 supplements derived from algae or fish oil may be taken into consideration. As with any supplement, it's best to speak with a healthcare provider.

Balance with Omega-6 Fatty Acids: It's essential for general health to maintain a balance between omega-3 and omega-6 fatty acid intake. Both kinds of fatty acids have different functions, and it's good to keep the right ratio.

4. Vitamin B Complex:
B vitamins, such as B12 and B6, are vital for neurotransmitter function and hormone control, two processes that are critical for many facets of general health, including sexual health. Overall sexual health and well-being are influenced by vitamin B complex, which plays roles in hormone regulation, neurotransmitter function, and energy metabolism. Maintaining ideal levels via a well-balanced diet and, when necessary, suitable supplements helps the body sustain sexual and reproductive vigor.

1. Hormone Regulation: The synthesis and regulation of hormones are mediated by B vitamins, particularly B12 and B6. The creation of sex hormones and other reproductive processes depend on hormonal balance. Sustaining adequate B vitamin levels facilitates the body's hormone regulation process. This is especially important when it comes to sex hormones that affect sexual health.

2. Neurotransmitter Function: The synthesis and control of neurotransmitters, such as dopamine and serotonin, are mediated by B vitamins. These neurotransmitters influence arousal, mood, and general mental health. The synthesis of neurotransmitters linked to mood control is facilitated by B vitamins. A healthy emotional state is necessary for a satisfying sexual encounter. B vitamin-influenced neurotransmitters are linked to pleasure and arousal. Sustaining sufficient levels facilitates these elements of supports these aspects of sexual health.

3. Energy Metabolism: The process of turning food into energy depends on B vitamins, which are essential to this process. Having enough energy is necessary for general vitality, which includes sexual endurance. B vitamins enhance energy metabolism, which raises general energy levels. For physical endurance and stamina during sexual engagement, this is advantageous.

Dietary Sources:
Meat, seafood, dairy products, leafy greens, and whole grains are just a few of the foods that contain B vitamins. Consuming these foods in a balanced diet helps increase B vitamin intake.

5. Magnesium

An essential element, magnesium influences many physiological processes that may have an impact on neuromuscular regulation, nerve transmission, and muscle function. Its function in these processes could have an impact on general sexual health and ejaculatory regulation. Magnesium may have an effect on ejaculatory control and general sexual health because of its role in muscle function, nerve transmission, and stress management. Maintaining ideal magnesium levels via a healthy diet and, if required, suitable supplementation promotes neuromuscular function and enhances libido.

1. Muscle Function: Both the contraction and relaxation of muscles depend on magnesium for healthy muscle function. Sufficient quantities of magnesium aid in controlling muscular tone and sensitivity. Sustaining ideal magnesium levels promotes muscle control, which is important for neuromuscular function in general and for controlling the pelvic muscles used in ejaculation in particular.

2. Nerve Transmission: Signaling and nerve transmission are two areas in which magnesium is involved. It aids in the effective transmission of

nerve impulses and the control of
neurotransmitters.
Enough magnesium is needed for the nervous
system to operate as it should. This is pertinent to
nerve transmission in general, which affects the
regulation of ejaculation.

3. Stress and Relaxation: Magnesium has the ability
to lower stress and increase relaxation. It affects
how the parasympathetic nervous system, which is
linked to relaxation, is activated. Stress
management may benefit from magnesium's
relaxing properties. Reducing stress has an impact
on ejaculatory control and overall sexual well-being.

-Dietary Sources: Leafy greens, legumes, nuts,
seeds, and whole grains are among the foods that
contain magnesium. Consuming magnesium is
facilitated by a diet that is well-balanced and
incorporates these sources.

Add-ons to Enhance Performance

1. L-arginine

An amino acid, L-arginine is an essential precursor
of nitric oxide. The vaginal area receives better
blood flow as a result of nitric oxide's ability to relax
blood vessels. This process could improve general
sexual performance and erection. Because

L-arginine stimulates the generation of nitric oxide, it helps vasodilate and increases blood flow. Both sexual performance and erectile function may benefit from this.

2. Ginseng Supplements

The plant renowned for its possible effects on sexual function is concentrated in ginseng supplements, especially those that contain Panax ginseng. These supplements may improve energy levels and blood flow, which may enhance overall sexual performance. Ginseng has long been thought to improve erotic activity. Supplements in concentrated forms are meant to offer reliable and powerful benefits.

3. Citrulline

Another amino acid that can boost the synthesis of nitric oxide is citrulline. Consequently, this encourages vasodilation and better blood flow. Supplementing with citrulline may enhance overall sexual performance and improve erectile function. Because citrulline aids in the synthesis of nitric oxide, blood vessels dilate and blood flow is improved. Sexual performance and erection function may benefit from this.

4. Comprehensive Multivitamin and Mineral Supplements

These supplements offer a wide range of nutrients that are vital for general health, including sexual wellness. For people whose sexual function may be affected by vitamin shortages, these supplements are helpful. Potential nutritional gaps can be filled by taking a well-balanced supplement, which guarantees the body gets the vitamins and minerals it needs for proper physiological performance, which includes components of sexual health.

Adhering to prescribed dosages is essential for the secure and efficient utilization of supplements. A healthcare provider should be consulted before beginning any supplements program.

Supplements can be helpful, but they work best when paired with a healthy lifestyle that includes stress reduction, regular exercise, and a balanced diet.

Chapter Six: Mastery through Practice

Gradual Progression in Sexual Activities

Developing confidence, control, and mastery in the area of intimacy can be achieved by a deliberate and strategic approach to gradual advancement in sexual activities. This approach aims to provide a supportive and positive sexual experience by acknowledging the interaction between physical and emotional variables. Building confidence, trust, and control in close relationships can be achieved with a deliberate and courteous approach to gradual sexual advancement. Partners can build a happy and supportive sexual encounter that stresses emotional connection and mutual enjoyment by first learning each other's comfort zones, then gradually introducing more stimulating elements.

Let's look at the salient features below:

1. Steep Advancement in Sexual Behaviors: A planned and conscious approach to building confidence, control, and mastery in the area of intimacy is the gradual escalation of sexual activities. In order to provide a happy and supportive sexual encounter, this approach recognizes the complex interplay between physical and emotional factors.

Building confidence, trust, and control in close relationships can be achieved with a deliberate and courteous approach to gradual sexual advancement. Partners can build a happy and supportive sexual encounter that stresses emotional connection and mutual enjoyment by first learning each other's comfort zones, then gradually introducing more stimulating elements.

This approach involves:

1. Knowing Your Personal Comfort Zones:
A thorough evaluation of each person's comfort zone is the first step in the process of progressive advancement. To discover one's own boundaries, desires, and intimacy-related worries, this requires introspection. A shared understanding must be established through open conversation with one's spouse. Building trust between partners involves recognizing and honoring each person's comfort zone. Building an atmosphere where people feel supported and protected while they progress is based on trust.

2. Building the Foundation with Less Demanding Activities: Less physically and emotionally taxing tasks are started to facilitate the process. This could include massages that are sensual, non-genital contact, or activities that emphasize emotional connection. The idea is to establish a foundation of security and confidence. Activities with lower demands lessen tension and the need to perform well. The goal of this first stage is to encourage relaxation so that a gradual and satisfying sexual encounter might occur.

3. Moving Up to Moderately Exciting Activities: Activities that are somewhat stimulating are added to the progression as comfort and confidence increase. During this stage, you might experiment with various erogenous zones, use mild arousal methods, and have more intimacy. Every step is made at a speed that suits both couples' comfort levels. Improving partners' emotional and physical connection is the main goal. This phase promotes mutual understanding and happiness by reinforcing the notion that sexual intimacy is a joint exploration.

4. Incorporating Stimulation and Genital Touch: Genital touch and stimulation are incorporated into the development, which starts with a foundation of

comfort and trust. With a focus on communication, permission, and the investigation of mutual enjoyment, this phase is undertaken deliberately. Performance becomes less important and more about mutual happiness. Activities between partners put an emphasis on intimacy, enjoyment, and progressively exploring each other's desires.

5. Exploring Sexual Intercourse: The introduction of sexual activity occurs when both partners are at ease and ready. At this point, the steady development has produced a setting where intimacy is valued and shared experiences are highlighted. The choice to have sex is determined by open communication and mutual consent. Open communication between partners guarantees a satisfying and consenting encounter.

6. Preserving a Helpful Environment: All the way through the process, the focus is on developing emotional bonding in addition to physical exploration. This all-encompassing strategy emphasizes the value of mutual closeness and understanding while reinforcing the notion that sexual mastery is a journey that transcends performance. No matter how big or small the progress is, praising and acknowledging it helps create a positive feedback loop. This method

promotes an attitude that emphasizes the continuous process of sexual mastery and discovery.

2. Starting Less Demanding Activities:
Starting a journey of steady sexual evolution begins with a deliberate entry into less physically and emotionally taxing practices.
A purposeful and fundamental step in the progressive growth of sexual activities is to begin with less strenuous actions. A mutually gratifying and encouraged sexual journey can be facilitated by partners creating a pleasant environment that emphasizes emotional connection, builds trust, fosters a sense of safety, and lays the framework for future exploration.
This thoughtful strategy creates the conditions for a satisfying and encouraging sexual encounter.

This important stage involves:

1. Establishing the Foundation: The process starts with intimate activities rather than intense ones. Sensual massages, non-genital contact, and other non-obtrusive physical forms of connection lay the groundwork for partners to become more responsive to one another. This phase's activities prioritize physical and emotional bonding above

instant genital stimulation. Through shared experiences, partners can better grasp each other's boundaries and wants.

2. Establishing Trust: Integrating and Communicating: There is a chance for candid discussion about expectations, comfort zones, and preferences during this first round. In order to create a mutual understanding, partners talk about their desires and boundaries. By partaking in less demanding activities, one can explore with another without feeling compelled to perform. As couples explore the path together and learn about each other's responses, this discovery helps to foster trust.

3. Establishing a Feeling of Security: Activities that require less effort are purposefully made to lessen tension and pressure to perform well. This stage creates a relaxed and safe environment where partners may express themselves without worrying about being judged. Partners concentrate on setting up a welcoming and suitable space for discovery. This entails things like maintaining a supportive environment through communication, maintaining privacy, and being aware of each other's emotional moods.

4. Building the Foundation for Further Development: The pursuits selected for this stage are baby steps toward experiences that are more exciting. With mindfulness, each step is taken to make sure both partners are at ease and prepared for the next stage. Creating a foundation of safety and trust creates a framework for comprehending boundaries. Couples learn to read each other's signs and cues regarding comfort and discomfort, which makes the process more cooperative and progressive.

3. Progressing to Mildly Stimulating Activities:

The next step in the slow development of sex is a deliberate shift to rather exhilarating encounters. Incremental steps that encourage more intimacy and investigation characterize this phase. Maintaining an open and transparent line of communication is crucial for creating a common understanding and strengthening emotional bonds. Increasing intimacy and exploration gradually and mindfully is necessary when moving on to somewhat exciting activities. Partners can build a joyful and shared sexual experience by taking little steps, discovering erogenous zones, using gentle arousal techniques, and keeping lines of communication open. This stage helps to maintain the growth of trust and emotional connection while laying the foundation for further investigation.

Now let's look at the essential elements of moving on to activities that are moderately stimulating:

1. Incremental Steps by: People are able to gradually increase their comfort levels if a base is laid in easier activities. Activities that are mildly arousing gradually build in intensity, letting partners discover new aspects of intimacy. The flow is adjusted to the tempo and tastes of each partner. Every action is done with awareness, making sure that the degree of stimulation corresponds with the comfort and preparedness of the people engaged.

2. Higher Degrees of Closeness: Part of the modestly exciting exercises involves partners exploring various erogenous zones. This can involve soft caresses, kisses, and touches in places that raise arousal. The goal is to strengthen the physical bond between couples and increase their comprehension of one another's reactions. Finding out what makes both of them happy and satisfied is possible at this point.

3. Calm Arousal Methods: Engaging in mildly arousing hobbies could involve trying out different gentle arousal methods. This could include methods that raise excitement without producing uncomfortable sensations—that is, preserving a balance that respects each partner's comfort levels. It's still crucial to have open lines of communication on preferences and limits. In order to create a climate of trust and cooperation, partners must obtain consent and make sure they are both prepared before introducing any new technique.

4. Expressing Feelings and Desires: It is crucial to maintain contact throughout this process. Partners communicate their needs, wants, and any worries they may have in an honest and open manner. This conversation facilitates a shared understanding and makes sure that both parties are in agreement. Partners can evaluate comfort levels and go through any necessary adjustments by checking in frequently before, during, and after these activities. An atmosphere that is accommodating and supportive is fostered by this constant contact.

4. Incorporating Touch and Stimulation of the Genitalia:

The growth of sexual activities necessitates the transition to genital touch and stimulation. A conscious strategy that prioritizes mutual agreement, exploration, and the progressive introduction of arousal is necessary during this phase. The goal is to foster a healthy sexual atmosphere where enjoyment is shared rather than gained via performance.

A mindful shift characterized by mutual agreement, exploration, and an emphasis on pleasure shared by both parties is required to incorporate genital touch and stimulation. This stage helps to establish a healthy sexual environment where understanding and connection are valued. Together, partners follow this path, creating a mutually fulfilling and exploratory experience.

Let's look at the essential elements of using genital stimulation and touch:

1. Intentional Change: Partners evaluate their comfort and preparedness levels prior to engaging in genital contact. In order to ensure a peaceful and deliberate shift, this phase calls for a shared awareness of each other's boundaries and desires.

During this change, partners keep lines of communication open to express their expectations, thoughts, and any potential worries. This constant communication creates a supportive and understanding environment.

2. Exploration and Mutual Consent: Couples approach genital contact with an open mind and an eagerness to learn. This stage enables both parties to find what makes them happy, which promotes a deeper comprehension of one another's needs. The emphasis is on mutual consent, with partners checking in and making sure that every move is appreciated. This thoughtful strategy strengthens the notion that the sexual journey is a shared experience and fosters trust.

3. Increasing Arousal Gradually: Arousal strategies are introduced gradually, emphasizing connection over performance. In order to prioritize the shared experience over individual expectations, partners experiment with approaches that increase intimacy and pleasure. This phase's pace is modified in accordance with each partner's comfort level and response. A positive and encouraging experience is promoted by taking gradual steps to ensure that the introduction of genital touch corresponds with the preparedness of individuals concerned.

4. Mutual Enjoyment as the Main Focus: In this phase, mutual enjoyment takes precedence over performance. By putting each other's happiness and contentment first, partners create a conducive atmosphere for a satisfying and happy sexual relationship. It is recommended that partners experiment in a responsive manner, modifying actions in response to cues and feedback. This adaptability guarantees that the experience is customized to the changing tastes and comfort levels of both people.

5. Exploring Sexual Intercourse:
Starting a sexual relationship is a big step in the development of sexual activity. This stage is characterized by careful scheduling planning and an emphasis on comfort and permission from both parties.

The last stage of the process is exploring sexual activity, which is characterized by constant communication, thoughtful timing, and mutual agreement. Couples make decisions together to make sure the encounter is agreeable, fulfilling, and compatible with each partner's comfort zone. This stage highlights the significance of the process in developing a satisfying and meaningful sexual connection.

The main facets of investigating sexual activity:

1. Timing Is Everything: The introduction of sexual activity happens at a speed that suits both partners' comfort levels and levels of readiness. The time is carefully selected to guarantee that people have reached the required degree of confidence, comfort, and trust. This stage's slow advancement helps to reduce anxiety and boost confidence. Since a foundation of trust has been built, it is a natural and supported step to introduce sexual activity.

2. Comfort and Mutual Consent: Couples keep lines of communication open on their thoughts, feelings, and any reservations they may have about having sex. This continuous conversation fosters a constructive and cooperative environment by reiterating a shared understanding. Partners check in with each other before, during, and after sexual activity to guarantee continued consent and comfort. By putting the needs of both parties first, this strategy promotes responsiveness and collaboration.

3. Deciding Together: Partners communicate their expectations and wants for sexual activity. By working together to make decisions, this approach makes sure that everyone is in agreement and

actively involved in the investigation of this new stage. Sexual relations is viewed as a collaborative discovery that prioritizes the bond between couples over performance. This kind of thinking promotes a supportive and pleasurable sexual experience.

4. A Harmonious and Fulfilling Experience: The earlier stages of the progressive evolution have prepared the environment for a pleasurable and consensual sex encounter. Couples rely on the closeness and trust they have built up over time. During sexual activity, partners maintain responsive communication, which enables them to adjust to each other's preferences and feedback. This flexibility improves the whole experience and strengthens the idea that sexual exploration is something that is done together.

6. Keeping a Helpful Environment: Maintaining a nurturing environment is essential to the entire process of sexual discovery and development. This continuous effort entails putting a strong emphasis on emotional connection, acknowledging accomplishments, and encouraging a holistic mindset that prioritizes intimacy over output.

Sustaining a supportive environment necessitates an ongoing dedication to emotional connection, progress celebration, and an appreciation of the sexual exploration path. Partners actively support an atmosphere that promotes development, flexible learning, and overall wellbeing. This methodical technique lays the groundwork for a satisfying and meaningful sexual relationship by reaffirming that sexual mastery is a shared and dynamic endeavor.

The essential elements of preserving a helpful environment include:

1. Prioritizing Emotional Bonding: The focus is still on encouraging emotional bonding in addition to physical discovery. Partners understand that achieving sexual mastery involves more than just performance; it also involves developing a stronger emotional link, mutual understanding, and shared intimacy. Vulnerability and open communication remain top priorities. When partners communicate their thoughts, feelings, and desires to one another, an atmosphere that fosters emotional connection and strengthens their relationship is created.

2. Recognizing Advancement: No matter how small, acknowledging and applauding progress creates a positive reinforcement loop. Partners who actively acknowledge and value one other's efforts cultivate a mindset that places a high importance on the continuous process of sexual discovery.
The collaborative quality of the sexual journey is strengthened when celebrating progress becomes a shared experience. Partners encourage one another's development, which adds to a feeling of fulfillment and success.

3. Mindset Shift: There is a mental change that prioritizes the trip over dwelling on one's perceived flaws. Partners know that sexual exploration is a dynamic process and that mastery is a journey rather than a destination. The environment promotes adaptive learning, in which partners modify their strategy in response to experiences and input. This adaptability fosters a nurturing atmosphere that promotes development and understanding amongst people.

4. Total Well-Being: The environment of support goes beyond the explicit sexual components of sex exploration. Partners value overall health, understanding that a satisfying sexual relationship is reliant on the interconnectedness of physical,

mental, and emotional well-being. Patience and resilience become essential elements of the encouraging environment. Partners are aware that obstacles could appear and that failures are a necessary part of learning. This knowledge encourages a resilient and patient method of exploring one's sexuality.

Building confidence, trust, and control through gradual advancement in sexual activities is a thoughtful and intentional strategy. Through the gradual integration of increasingly complicated aspects into less difficult activities, people can develop a healthy sexual experience that places an emphasis on mutual pleasure and emotional connection. This path to sexual mastery requires open communication, mutual trust, and celebration of accomplishments.

Methods to Postpone Ejaculation

It is possible to improve control and mastery over one's sexual impulses by using a variety of ways to postpone ejaculation. Enhancing awareness, controlling arousal, and fostering a more fulfilling and regulated sexual experience are the goals of these strategies. Here is a thorough examination of two important techniques:

1. Stop-start Technique:

The behavioral strategy called the stop-start method aims to improve control over ejaculation. The stop-start approach is predicated on the notion that arousal can be lowered and ejaculation can be postponed by stopping sexual stimulation. People try to control their level of excitement and avoid an early climax by purposefully pausing during sexual engagement at specific times.

Practice Steps:

1. Starting Sexual Activity: Start having sex like you usually would, whether it be through foreplay or sexual contact.

2. Strategic Pauses: As the climax approaches, purposefully reduce or stop all stimulation. This is an intentional pause to allow for a reduction in excitement.

3. Subsiding Arousal:** Concentrate on letting arousal drop during the break. To regain control and avoid ejaculating too soon, this step is crucial.

4. Continuing the Activity: Resume your sexual activity after your arousal has decreased. To extend the sexual experience, repeat the procedure as needed.

Advantages:

1. Enhanced Control:By giving people a useful technique to stop the climax from building, the procedure improves their ability to regulate their arousal levels.

2. Increased Awareness: Using the stop-start method makes one more conscious of their arousal patterns and makes it easier to spot the cues that indicate ejaculation.

3. Versatility: This method encourages candid communication and teamwork and can be modified for usage during paired or solitary sexual activities.

When used regularly, the stop-start technique aids in the development of ejaculatory control and a more satisfying sexual experience.

2. Squeezing Technique:

Pressure is applied to the base of the penis just prior to reaching the point of climax in the squeezing technique, a behavioral strategy used to postpone ejaculation. Using physical intervention to lower arousal, this therapy seeks to halt the body's normal march toward ejaculation.

Practice Steps:
1. Start your typical sexual activities, such as intimate kissing or foreplay.

2. Indicate to your partner or give yourself a hard grip on the base of your penis as soon as you feel like you are getting close to the breaking point.

3. Hold the pressure for approximately thirty seconds. An arousal reduction is possible at this time.

4. Resuming sexual activity is advised after letting go of the pressure. If necessary, repeat the procedure.

Advantages:
1. The squeezing technique is a useful tactic during sexual interactions by presenting a prompt and straightforward way to interfere when ejaculation is approaching.
2. By adding a tactile component, the method raises people's consciousness of the bodily experiences connected to arousal.
3. By actively using the squeezing technique, partners can enhance a cooperative and encouraging sex experience.

The squeezing technique and the stop-start method both benefit from frequent practice, either by yourself or with a partner. When used consistently, people can become more aware of their arousal patterns and improve their capacity to postpone ejaculation.

Incorporating these strategies requires open communication between partners. talking about individual preferences, comfort zones, and collectively improving the practice

Reinforcing Positive Habits

1. A comprehensive approach to sexual mastery that emphasizes the development of attitudes and actions that lead to a meaningful and pleasurable sexual experience is called "reinforcing positive habits." This entails deliberate actions, dialogue techniques, and mental adjustments that promote a healthy sexual environment. Now let's examine the essential elements of strengthening constructive habits:

2. Establishing Reasonable Expectations: Recognizing that sexual mastery is a skill that must be learned is a necessary step in reinforcing healthy habits. Realistic expectations encourage patience

and an understanding that change requires time and work from both partners and individuals. Appreciating small victories instead of concentrating only on goals fosters a positive outlook. Acknowledging and valuing accomplishments, regardless of size, helps one feel accomplished and provides drive for further development.

3. Retaining a Positive Attitude: Positive behaviors must be reinforced by embracing a growth mentality. This entails seeing obstacles as chances for growth and learning. Couples actively participate in the path to sexual mastery with an open mind and a readiness to change. Resilience is necessary to reinforce healthy behaviors. Partners accept that obstacles may arise, but rather than seeing them as failures, they see them as chances to grow and modify their approaches in order to achieve success in the future.

4. Establishing a Helpful Environment: Emotional safety is given priority in a supportive setting. People can freely express their feelings and ideas without worrying about being judged, fostering an environment where being vulnerable is welcomed. Recognizing when further assistance is required is part of reinforcing beneficial habits. Partners advise

obtaining expert assistance to investigate comprehensive solutions and improve the learning process, such as speaking with therapists or healthcare specialists.

5. Acknowledging and Reinforcing Mutual Satisfaction: Recognizing that mutual satisfaction is a shared obligation between couples is a necessary step in reinforcing beneficial habits. This cooperative strategy encourages a sense of oneness and teamwork in achieving a satisfying sexual experience. Partners actively show gratitude for one another's endeavors and contributions to the common goal of achieving sexual mastery. Positive reinforcement like this fortifies the emotional bond and inspires further improvement.

Chapter Seven: Overcoming Psychological Barriers in Premature Ejaculation

Taking Care of Performance Anxiety

A multimodal strategy is needed to address performance anxiety in premature ejaculation:

1. Understanding Triggers:
One of the most important steps in treating performance anxiety related to early ejaculation is identifying triggers. People can create successful strategies for getting past psychological obstacles by recognizing specific triggers, encouraging open communication, looking for therapeutic solutions, using gradual exposure tactics, including mindfulness practices, and involving the partner.

1. Identifying particular elements that lead to performance anxiety is necessary in order to comprehend triggers in the context of premature ejaculation. Among them are

1. People may feel anxious because they worry that their partner will judge them. In order to address this trigger, it is important to promote open communication and establish a safe space where

both partners may freely express their wants and worries.

2. Anxiety might be triggered by past negative sexual encounters. To reduce anxiety and foster a positive outlook, it is crucial to acknowledge and process these events, either on your own or with assistance from a partner or therapist. Individuals can address the underlying causes of performance anxiety and move toward a more confident and gratifying sexual experience by identifying these triggers, which lays the groundwork for focussed intervention.

2. Talk with your partner:
Yes, managing stress related to performance requires having an honest and open dialogue with your partner. The reason is because the establishment of a supportive atmosphere is facilitated by the sharing of worries, anxieties, and expectations. That way, each partner may do their share to foster an environment that fosters empathy and understanding. Partners who make a cooperative effort can effectively handle and control stress associated to performance. In response to the difficulties brought on by early ejaculation, cooperative efforts strengthen the bond and foster a sense of unity.

Partners' understanding is fostered through communication. Open communication about issues helps people understand one another's viewpoints, which improves empathy and fosters a closer bond. The cooperative method of handling stress associated to performance fortifies the emotional connection between partners. Collaborating establishes a mutual path towards conquering obstacles, strengthening the bond within the partnership.

3. Therapeutic Interventions:

Therapeutic interventions provide a multimodal approach to address performance anxiety in overcoming psychological barriers related to premature ejaculation. These interventions include counseling, cognitive-behavioral therapy, mindfulness practices, gradual exposure therapy, pharmacological support, and communication skills training.

1. Sex therapy and counseling: A private, secure setting is offered by professional counseling or sex therapy for the purpose of exploring and treating performance anxiety. Counselors can help people understand the underlying reasons of anxiety, provide psychoeducation, and suggest coping mechanisms.

2. Cognitive-Behavioral Therapy (CBT): CBT is a popular therapy strategy that aims to recognize and alter unfavorable thinking patterns and behavior patterns. CBT assists people in managing their anxiety, reframing their negative thoughts, and adopting more positive attitudes about sexual performance when it comes to premature ejaculation.

3. Relaxation and Mindfulness Methods: Therapeutic methods may include the integration of mindfulness techniques, such as deep breathing, meditation, and relaxation exercises. These methods lessen worry, increase resilience, and support mental health in general.

4. Gradual Exposure Therapy: Gradual exposure entails methodically and gradually exposing oneself to anxiety-inducing events. This method enables people to gradually become less sensitive to performance-related stress in the setting of premature ejaculation.

5. Pharmacological Support:.To treat psychological reasons contributing to premature ejaculation, medical practitioners may occasionally administer drugs or topical anesthetics. The goals of these

therapy are to improve ejaculatory control and reduce anxiety.

6. Training in Communication Skills: Therapists may concentrate on enhancing a client's ability to communicate with a partner as well as with themselves. Good communication creates a helpful sexual environment by assisting people in expressing their expectations, worries, and wishes.

4. Techniques for Gradual Exposure:
An organized and scientifically supported method of treating performance anxiety in premature ejaculation is provided by gradual exposure strategies. People can desensitize to stresses by methodically confronting anxiety-inducing circumstances with a therapist's help. This will help them progressively gain confidence and improve their ability to control their ejaculation.

Here is a rundown:

1. Knowing Your Personal Triggers: It's crucial to pinpoint the precise triggers producing performance anxiety prior to starting the progressive exposure method. This could involve worries about pleasing a partner, dread of being judged, or bad memories from the past.

2. Building a Hierarchy of Situations that Trigger Anxiety: Therapists collaborate with clients to develop a hierarchy of scenarios that cause different degrees of anxiety. These circumstances are ordered from least to most likely to cause anxiety.

3. Systematic Desensitization: The person is progressively exposed to events ranked from least anxiety-inducing to most anxiety-inducing. Over time, greater comfort and confidence are made possible by the regulated and encouraging setting in which this exposure takes place.

4. Progressive Steps: The person gradually advances to increasingly difficult scenarios as they become proficient in handling less anxiety-inducing ones. This methodical process reduces overpowering emotions and fosters a sense of accomplishment.

5. Incorporating Spouse Involvement: A supportive spouse may participate in the gradual exposure process. This cooperative strategy encourages candid dialogue and teamwork in reducing stress associated with performance.

6. Repetition and Reinforcement: Positive experiences are reinforced by regular and repeated exposure to anxiety-inducing circumstances. This repetition fosters resilience in the face of adversity and helps change unfavorable connections.

5. Mindfulness Techniques:
The management of performance anxiety resulting from premature ejaculation is greatly aided by mindfulness methods.
An effective and approachable method of treating performance anxiety is through mindfulness techniques. People can overcome the difficulties associated with premature ejaculation by cultivating calmness, lowering worry, and strengthening emotional fortitude.

1. Using Mindfulness Techniques: Mindfulness entails practicing acceptance of oneself without judgment and present-moment awareness. Anxiety management techniques include deep breathing, mindfulness exercises, and meditation that can be incorporated into everyday routines.

2. Encouraging Calm: Mindfulness exercises are beneficial in encouraging calm. Exercises that involve deep breathing, for instance, trigger the body's relaxation response, which lowers

physiological arousal linked to performance anxiety.

3. Reduction of Anxiety: Mindfulness practices assist people in seeing their thoughts and feelings without being overcome by them. By raising knowledge of this, anxiety levels may be lowered and a more balanced viewpoint on sexual experiences may result.

4. Building Sturdiness: Maintaining a regular mindfulness practice helps people become more emotionally resilient. By cultivating an attitude of acceptance and non-reactivity, people become more resilient to pressures, especially worries about their performance.

5. Integration into Everyday Existence: The versatility of mindfulness activities in day-to-day living is their charm. These practices, which include mindful breathing exercises, brief meditation sessions, and moment-to-moment mindfulness, can be easily incorporated into everyday routines.

Increasing Self-Esteem and Confidence

When it comes to controlling premature ejaculation, positive reinforcement is an essential component of self-esteem and confidence building. A positive feedback loop is created by recognizing and appreciating tiny victories, which helps one develop a more positive self-image. Acknowledging one's own talents and accomplishments gives people a sense of self-satisfaction and boosts their confidence in their capacity to manage and enhance their sexual experiences. This optimistic outlook serves as the cornerstone for developing resilience and a more assured strategy for dealing with early ejaculation.

1. Setting Realistic Goals:
In order to overcome premature ejaculation, it is essential to set realistic goals in order to increase self-esteem and confidence.

Understanding Individual Progress: Every person's journey is different, and recognizing personal growth is a necessary part of setting realistic goals. A methodical strategy to controlling premature ejaculation is made possible by setting clear, attainable goals.

Steer clear of unrealistic expectations: Performance anxiety may be exacerbated by unrealistic expectations. People can feel accomplished without putting too much pressure on themselves if they create objectives that are difficult yet doable.

Remembering Little Steps Forward: A positive outlook is promoted by acknowledging and appreciating tiny but meaningful improvements. This encouraging feedback helps to gradually develop confidence by reiterating the notion that development is constant.

Partner Involvement: Discussing objectives with a helpful companion might make the trip more cooperative. Positive and encouraging sexual environment and understanding are fostered by open discussion about mutual objectives.

In the context of treating premature ejaculation, setting realistic goals is a proactive and powerful way to enhance confidence and self-esteem. It is consistent with the notion that growth occurs gradually and that every accomplishment adds to a resilient and optimistic outlook on life.

2. Guidance and Assistance:

Managing premature ejaculation is one area in which professional therapy is extremely important for enhancing self-esteem and confidence.

1. Safe Exploration: Individuals seeking assistance with confidence issues associated with premature ejaculation can find a secure and private setting in counseling. Talking with an experienced professional about your worries, thoughts, and experiences can provide insightful advice.

2. Behavioral and Cognitive Strategies: To reframe unfavorable thought patterns linked to performance anxiety, therapists frequently utilize cognitive-behavioral techniques. This could entail creating more constructive self-talk, recognizing and addressing harmful beliefs, and creating coping techniques.

3. Capabilities for Communication:* Therapy sessions can improve a person's ability to communicate, making it easier for them to convey their wants, anxieties, and expectations. An atmosphere that is encouraging of sexual activity is fostered by enhanced communication, which helps to improve understanding between couples.

4. Personalized Guidance: Individualized advice from therapists is based on each person's unique needs and experiences. Because of this tailored approach, the techniques used are certain to support the person's objectives for increasing self-worth and confidence.

5. All-Around Wellness: Together with more general issues of mental health, counseling addresses the unique difficulties associated with early ejaculation. Holistic approaches to confidence building include techniques for stress, anxiety, and general mental health management.

Counseling Methods for Mental Well-Being

A comprehensive strategy is needed to explore therapeutic therapies for mental well-being in the context of controlling premature ejaculation:

1. Sex therapy and counseling: Counselors and sex therapists that specialize in early ejaculation offer specific advice. In order to improve mental health, this may entail addressing psychological issues, investigating communication tactics, and applying behavioral approaches.

Helping people understand the psychological implications of premature ejaculation lowers

anxiety and encourages a proactive approach to managing the illness.
Partners participate in sex therapy frequently, which promotes candid conversation and teamwork. An increased level of understanding and support arises when a partner is involved in the therapy process.

2. Mindfulness and Relaxation Techniques: The best ways to deal with stress and anxiety are through deep breathing exercises, meditation, and mindfulness. The psychological elements that lead to early ejaculation are lessened by these methods, which encourage mental serenity.
Remaining in the present moment and being more conscious of one's body language are two benefits of practicing mindfulness. Control of ejaculation may benefit from this heightened consciousness.

3. Medication and Pharmacological Support In certain situations, medical practitioners may recommend drugs or topical anesthetics to treat underlying psychological issues. Premature ejaculation is the goal of these therapies, which may necessitate consultation to determine eligibility and possible side effects. Healthcare providers perform a thorough examination to learn about the patient's

medical history, any contraindications, and preferences before writing a prescription.

A comprehensive approach to controlling psychological variables linked to early ejaculation and fostering general mental well-being involves incorporating psychotherapy, mindfulness exercises, and, when required, pharmaceutical help.

Chapter Eight: Maintaining Long-Term Success

It takes consistent work and tactics to manage premature ejaculation over the long term. Maintaining a healthy lifestyle with regular exercise, stress reduction, hydration, balanced diet, and thoughtful food selections all have a major role in the ongoing reduction of premature ejaculation. Over time, these techniques establish a comprehensive basis for improved sexual function and general well-being.

Strategies for Continued Improvement

1. Changes to Lifestyle:
Maintaining a healthy lifestyle as a top priority is essential for long-term success in controlling early ejaculation. This is an in-depth conversation:

1. Modifications to Lifestyle: It's crucial to keep eating a diet high in vital nutrients. The balance of hormones is supported by nutrients including zinc, vitamin D, and omega-3 fatty acids, which promote reproductive health in general. Your diet will be nutrient-dense if you prioritize whole, unprocessed foods.

2. Frequent Exercise: Regular exercise has a positive impact on general fitness and cardiovascular health. Increased blood flow from cardiovascular activity improves erectile function and has a good impact on ejaculatory control. Strength training activities are added to support physical endurance.

3. Stress Management: It is imperative to consistently apply stress management strategies. Prolonged stress can have a negative impact on nervous system function and hormone balance, which might lead to early ejaculation. Effective stress management strategies include regular exercise, mindfulness exercises, and relaxation methods.

4. Hydration: Sufficient hydration is still essential for general health, including erotic activity. Fatigue brought on by dehydration might affect energy levels and performance. Sustaining adequate hydration on a regular basis promotes physiological functions essential for healthy sexual functioning.

5. Reducing Sugar and Processed Food Intake: It takes dedication to cut back on added sugars and processed foods. Diets heavy in these components may alter the balance of hormones and cause

metabolic problems and obesity. Prioritizing complete, unprocessed diets promotes both sexual and overall wellness.

6. Moderate Intake of Alcohol: It's best to continue drinking alcohol in moderation. Overindulgence in alcohol can affect sexual function and neurological system function. Regular moderation improves ejaculatory control and promotes general health.

2. Keeping lines of communication open with your partner is essential to figuring out how to handle early ejaculation.
Regular check-ins, expressing feelings, active listening, collaborative decision-making, adaptability, positive reinforcement, and swift settlement of issues are all necessary to maintain open communication practices. These procedures set the stage for a cooperative and encouraging relationship that will last the duration of managing premature ejaculation.

Communication Techniques
1. Timely Check-Ins: Plan frequent times to talk about your thoughts, feelings, and any changes you've made to your strategy. By encouraging continuous communication, these check-ins make

sure that both partners are aware of each other's wants and worries.

2. Promote honest communication of any feelings you may have about the trip. By sharing both happy and difficult experiences, a safe space is created where empathy and understanding of one another's viewpoints can grow.

3. Active Listening: Make an effort to pay attention throughout conversations. This is paying close attention to what your spouse says and making an effort to get their point of view without passing judgment right away. Mutual understanding and a closer bond are fostered by active listening.

4. Collaborative Decision-Making: Treat the treatment of premature ejaculation as a team endeavor. Whether you are making adjustments to procedures, investigating new approaches, or consulting a professional, involve your partner in the decision-making process. Making decisions together strengthens a sense of unity.

5. Modifications and Adaptability: Remain flexible to adapt to each partner's changing requirements and preferences. Your capacity to be flexible shows

that you are adaptive and dedicated to coming up with solutions that work for all parties.

6. Positive Reinforcement: Highlight achievements and satisfying encounters. Recognizing accomplishments, no matter how minor, promotes a pleasant environment and a constant improvement mindset.

7.Addressing Concerns: As soon as an issue comes up, take immediate action. Proactively addressing difficulties stops unsolved problems from building up, which strengthens and fortifies a partnership.

3. Managing premature ejaculation requires ongoing education. Maintaining current knowledge, getting advice from experts, using learning materials, attending seminars, and being a part of encouraging groups are all part of ongoing education. Your ability to adjust and improve your methods for handling early ejaculation is enhanced by this dedication to lifelong learning.

Methods of Ongoing Education

1. Continuous Learning: Proactively look for information about recent advancements, scientific discoveries, and prevention techniques for early ejaculation. Keeping yourself informed gives you the tools to investigate other methods and approaches.

2. Expert Advice: To stay current on the most recent findings and suggestions, speak with medical experts, sex therapists, or other specialists. Receiving information that is precise, supported by evidence, and catered to your individual needs is certain when you seek professional guidance.

4. Educational Resources: Make use of trustworthy educational materials, such as books, articles, and websites devoted to sexual health. These resources offer helpful information and insightful analysis on a variety of premature ejaculation-related topics.

5. Workshops and Conferences: Participate in webinars, seminars, or workshops on relationship dynamics and sexual health. By taking part in these events, one can meet specialists, engage in interactive learning, and share experiences with others going through similar struggles.

6. Help for the Community: Participating in local or online communities centered around sexual health can help to promote peer-to-peer learning. A more comprehensive grasp of managing premature ejaculation is achieved through participating in conversations, exchanging experiences, and learning from the experiences of others.

7. Modification of Approaches: Be willing to modify your tactics as fresh information becomes available. By learning continuously, you can adjust your strategy in light of new information.

4. In order to successfully manage premature ejaculation over the long term, you must keep seeking professional advice. Here's a detailed analysis of this tactic:

4. Professional Guidance: Ongoing professional supervision entails timely resolution of new issues, frequent check-ins, therapeutic assistance, medication management, adherence to lifestyle advice, and knowledge of novel solutions. This method guarantees continuous assistance and modifications based on your changing requirements as you navigate the process of controlling early ejaculation.

1. Plan on seeing your doctor on a frequent basis to address any changes or worries you may have about ejaculating too soon, as well as to monitor your general health. Maintaining regular contact guarantees that any underlying health issues are dealt with right away.

2. Consider continuing to attend frequent appointments with your sex therapist or counselor even after you start to see results. A structured setting for addressing psychological issues and reinforcing healthy behaviors is offered via ongoing therapy assistance.

3. If you have been provided any drugs or topical treatments, follow the indicated course of action and keep in regular contact with your healthcare practitioner. Medication or dose modifications could be necessary based on your progress and any changes in health.

4. Keep up with the lifestyle advice given by medical professionals. Including these routines—whether they have to do with nutrition, physical activity, or stress reduction—improves general well-being and may have a favorable effect on ejaculatory control.

5. Keep up with any new therapies or interventions that may be developed in the field of sexual health. Your healthcare professional may advise you on the most recent choices, making sure that your strategy stays thorough and compliant with research-proven methods.

6. Discuss any new issues or problems as soon as possible with your healthcare professional. By keeping lines of communication open, you can make timely changes to your management plan and avoid future setbacks.

7. A person's sexual health may be impacted by changes in their relationships, employment, or way of life. Talk to your healthcare professional about any big changes so you may adjust your tactics.

Incorporating Techniques into Daily Life

1. Mindfulness Practices

The benefits of regulating premature ejaculation are extended when mindfulness practices are integrated into daily living. Living mindfully helps people handle stress better, communicate better in relationships, be more flexible when things change, and develop a body-mind connection. This all-encompassing strategy promotes long-term wellbeing and sexual health.

1. Adopting a Mindful Lifestyle: Include mindfulness in all aspects of your daily life. Incorporate brief mindfulness exercises, such deliberate moments of awareness or concentrated breathing exercises, into your daily routine.

2. Stress Management: Apply mindfulness practices to control anxiety and stress in day-to-day circumstances. Whenever you encounter difficulties, pause mindfully, breathe deeply, and focus on the here and now. Proactively managing stress can enhance one's mental health in general.

3. Connection and Communication:Apply attention to all of your social encounters, particularly romantic ones. During interactions, try to be really present and engage in active listening. This encourages closer ties and makes the atmosphere more sympathetic and helpful, even in close relationships.

4. Resolution of Conflicts: Being able to address confrontations with composure and focus is a skill of mindful life. When there is a disagreement, communicate mindfully, trying to grasp the other person's point of view instead of responding hastily.

5. Adaptability and Sturdiness: Living with mindfulness promotes adaptability and perseverance in the face of life's changes. Develop a flexible mindset that enables you to react calmly to changing situations. This flexibility includes incorporating methods for controlling early ejaculation.

6. Making Conscienceuous Decisions: Incorporate awareness into your decision-making. You can make decisions about your early ejaculation management and other aspects of your life that support your overall well-being by approaching choices with purposeful awareness.

7. Whole Perspective: Living mindfully highlights the relationship between the mind and body. This holistic approach recognizes the connection between mental health and physical experiences, which is consistent with the comprehensive treatments for treating premature ejaculation.

8. Trigger Awareness: Being mindful makes it easier to identify stress or anxiety-inducing triggers in both social and private contexts. Proactively managing these triggers is made possible by this increased awareness, which promotes overall emotional balance.

9. Exercises in Mindfulness: Mindfulness in Daily Life:* Develop an attitude of everyday mindfulness in addition to targeted mindfulness exercises. Take part in activities mindfully, enjoying every second of them. This method makes life richer and more satisfying on a daily basis.

Thankfulness Practice: As part of your mindful lifestyle, develop a thankfulness practice. Express your thankfulness for the good things in your life on a regular basis. This exercise improves one's ability to think positively and supports mental and emotional health in general.

2. Physical Fitness Routine

Keeping up a physical fitness regimen that includes strength training, aerobics, and pelvic floor exercises is essential to integrating methods into everyday life. This all-encompassing method promotes general health and wellbeing in addition to ejaculatory control. Consistent, regular work develops good habits that improve mental and physical health.

1. Exercise for the Heart: Include aerobic exercises in your regimen, such swimming, cycling, or jogging. Participating in these exercises promotes blood circulation, cardiovascular health, and

general stamina. Include cardiovascular activities in your everyday routine. Think about commuting by bicycle, walking briskly, or using the stairs. These decisions support long-term cardiovascular health, which enhances control over ejaculation.

2. Strength Training: Keep up a regular strength training regimen that includes bodyweight or weightlifting workouts. This supports general physical fitness and stamina by improving muscular tone and strength. Include strength exercise in your regular routine. During breaks, move household items, do bodyweight exercises, or have brief strength-training sessions. These modest but regular efforts add up to long-term fitness.

3. Exercises for the Pelvic Floor: Set aside a certain amount of time to perform pelvic floor exercises, such Kegels. Frequent exercise improves ejaculatory control by strengthening the pelvic floor muscles. Include these workouts in your everyday routine for long-term advantages. Make notes or associate pelvic floor exercises with routines you already follow, such as brushing your teeth. By creating a schedule, you can make sure that these workouts become a regular and organic part of your day.

4. Complete Fitness: The physical fitness regimen integrates muscle strength, pelvic floor stability, and cardiovascular health in a comprehensive approach to wellness. This all-encompassing approach is consistent with the multimodal management of premature ejaculation.

5. Enduring Advantages: You are making an investment in your long-term health by including these activities into your everyday routine. Maintaining a regular physical fitness level promotes a healthier and more active lifestyle by supporting both general well-being and ejaculatory control.

6. The Mind-Body Link: Exercise regimens for physical fitness support a robust mind-body connection. You're building a stronger bond between your physical and emotional wellness when you work out to improve your cardiovascular health and muscle strength.

7. Progress and Regularity: Including these workouts in your regular routine encourages consistency and steady advancement. Whether it's going the additional mile or stepping up the intensity of your strength exercise, recognize and celebrate your accomplishments.

Regular exercise becomes ingrained in the habit thanks to this positive reinforcement.

3. Good Eating Practices

One of the most important aspects of implementing methods into daily life is maintaining a nutrient-rich diet that emphasizes hormonal balance and cardiovascular health. Good eating practices enhance general wellbeing, have a good impact on sexual function, and promote a wholistic approach to healthcare. Consciously choosing food has long-term advantages that go beyond improving a person's ability to conceive, supporting a happier, better living.

1. Diet Rich in Nutrients:. Make eating a varied, well-balanced diet a priority. Add entire grains, fruits, veggies, lean meats, and healthy fats to your diet. This well-rounded strategy supplies vital vitamins and minerals to promote general wellness. Try a variety of foods to guarantee a range of nutrients. To encourage the best possible nutritional intake, choose whole grains, a variety of protein sources, and vibrant veggies.

2. Vital Components: Make sure the vital components in your diet promote hormonal equilibrium. Zinc, vitamin D, and omega-3 fatty

acids are among the nutrients that are important for hormone balance and general reproductive health.

Hormonal activity depends on an adequate protein intake. Incorporate sources such as dairy, legumes, plant-based proteins, and lean meats into your diet.

3. Health Circulatory System: Make dietary choices that support heart health. This includes foods that are low in saturated fats, high in heart-healthy fats (found in nuts, avocados, and olive oil), and high in fiber (such whole grains and legumes). Maintaining adequate hydration is crucial for heart health. Water consumption should be sufficient throughout the day to maintain general body functions.

4. Reduce Sugar and Processed Foods: Limit your consumption of highly processed foods, which can have high concentrations of harmful fats, additives, and preservatives. For best nutrition, choose whole, minimally processed meals. In your diet, cut back on additional sugars. Consuming too much sugar might worsen general health and aggravate inflammation. Select naturally occurring sweeteners, like fruits, where necessary.

5. Remain Hydrated: Many body processes, such as metabolism and circulation, depend on getting

enough water. To keep yourself properly hydrated during the day, make it a practice to drink water frequently.

6. Whole Well-Being:.Nutritional Influence on Health: Including good eating practices is consistent with a wholistic approach to wellness. Foods high in nutrients promote mental and physical wellness, which in turn enhances sexual performance. A long-term investment in general health is the establishment of healthy eating habits. Maintaining a healthy diet over time offers long-term advantages such as increased vitality, better mood, and optimal physiological processes.

7. Conscious Consumption: By observing your body's signals of hunger and fullness, cultivate mindful eating habits. Eating mindfully cultivates a more positive connection with food, enhancing contentment and general health.

8. Educational Awareness: Make educated decisions by keeping up to date on the nutritional value of foods. Having knowledge about how food choices affect cardiovascular health and hormone balance gives people the ability to put their bodies first.

A comprehensive strategy that incorporates lifestyle strategies, regular practice of techniques, continuous assessment, and adaptation is necessary to maintain long-term effectiveness in managing premature ejaculation. People can encourage ongoing progress and maintain favorable results over time by continuing to be proactive and adaptable.

Conclusions

Recap of Key Techniques

Many different approaches have been investigated for handling the process of controlling premature ejaculation. The physical and psychological effects of premature ejaculation can be effectively addressed with a variety of techniques, ranging from mindfulness and relaxation exercises to communication practices, from moderate sexual activity development to therapeutic approaches for mental well-being. Individuals are given a comprehensive approach to ejaculatory control through the utilization of a wide range of techniques, such as supplements, critical nutrients, and herbal therapies.

1. Mindfulness and Relaxation Exercises: Methods like progressive muscle relaxation and mindfulness meditation provide people the skills they need to manage their anxiety, become more self-aware, and relax, all of which are fundamental to treating premature ejaculation.

2. Breathing Techniques for Control: The 4-7-8 technique, box breathing, deep diaphragmatic breathing, and synchronized breathing with a partner are effective ways to lower excitement, relax the nervous system, and improve overall control during sexual encounters.

3. Visualization and Mental Conditioning: Techniques for reshaping thought patterns, lowering anxiety, and creating a positive mental association with sexual experiences include mental conditioning scripts, cue-controlled relaxation, and visualization-based desensitization.

4. Herbal Treatments for Sexual Wellness: Tribulus Terrestris, Maca Root, Ashwagandha, Ginseng, Horny Goat Weed, and Ginkgo Biloba are examples of natural remedies. These herbs are thought to have beneficial effects on blood circulation, hormone balance, and sexual function.

5. Essential Nutrients and Their Role: Zinc, magnesium, vitamin B complex, vitamin D, and omega-3 fatty acids are important for neurotransmitter function, cardiovascular health, and hormone regulation.

6. Supplements to Support Performance: L-arginine, multivitamin/mineral supplements, ginseng supplements, and citrulline provide further support for enhanced blood flow, nitric oxide production, and general sexual health.

7. Incremental Advancement in Sexual Behaviors: Building confidence, trust, and control gradually is facilitated by a staged strategy that begins with less difficult activities and advances to increasingly engaging encounters. It places a focus on sharing enjoyment and exploring together with a partner.

8. Techniques for Delaying Ejaculation: The squeezing technique and the stop-start approach are useful ways to postpone ejaculation, giving people useful tools to control arousal and improve controlling ejaculation.

9. Reinforcing Positive Habits: Building an emotional connection, appreciating progress, keeping a positive outlook, encouraging open communication, and having reasonable expectations are all important aspects of reinforcing positive habits for sexual mastery.

10. Overcoming Barriers Related to Psychology: It takes knowledge of triggers, careful exposure, and honest dialogue with a partner to address performance anxiety. Positive reinforcement, realistic goal-setting, and seeking out therapy treatments are all important components of boosting self-esteem and confidence. Counseling, mindfulness training, and medicine when needed are further strategies for promoting mental health.

By acknowledging the connections between physical, psychological, and relational aspects of sexual well-being, these essential strategies come together to provide a whole strategy for treating premature ejaculation.

Encouragement for a Fulfilling Sexual Life

Adopting the techniques covered in this extensive manual is a commitment to building a satisfying sexual life, not just a solution for early ejaculation. People can achieve sexual mastery through establishing positive habits, being in constant communication with their partner, and integrating mindfulness into their daily experiences. A deeper connection is cultivated by placing a strong emphasis on comprehension, empathy, and shared responsibility with a partner. This improves the quality of intimate relationships generally as well as sexual fulfillment.

It is crucial to see this path as a chance for personal development and discovery, understanding that sexual mastery is a dynamic and ever-evolving process. A good outlook, realistic expectations, and acknowledging accomplishments are all factors in fostering a favorable sexual self-image. The strategies provided are not rigid rules but adaptable tools that individuals can tailor to their unique needs and preferences, creating a personalized approach to sexual well-being.

1. Celebrating Progress: No matter how little a milestone may be, it should be recognized and celebrated. Every advancement—whether it is in technique mastery, partner communication, or general well-being—is a success that should be acknowledged.

2. Embracing the Learning Process: Recognize that gaining sexual expertise requires learning. Approach every encounter with curiosity and an open mind, and practice self-compassion. Accepting the learning process promotes a growth-oriented, optimistic outlook.

3. Building a Stronger Bond with Your Spouse: The process of getting over early ejaculation offers a chance to strengthen your bond with your spouse on a physical and emotional level. An open line of communication, reciprocal assistance, and joint discovery lead to a deeper and more fulfilling partnership.

4. Adjusting to Changing Needs: Understand that requirements and situations might alter over time. Remain aware of your partner's and your own changing tastes. Sustaining satisfaction requires a readiness to change and investigate novel ideas.

5. Centering on General Well-Being: Recall that overall wellbeing and sexual health are closely related. Maintain your focus on leading a healthy lifestyle, which includes stress reduction, frequent exercise, and a balanced diet. Sexual function is positively impacted by a holistic approach to wellbeing.

6. Seeking Expert Assistance When Necessary: Do not hesitate to seek expert assistance if problems continue or if you have any new concerns. Professionals can provide specialized solutions to address particular needs and problems, whether through counseling, therapy, or medical guidance.

7. Developing Confidence in Intimacy: As you put tactics and methods into practice, concentrate on developing personal confidence. Have a positive self-image and recognize that having sex is a personal, unique experience that may be very gratifying.

8. Maintaining a Positive Outlook: Remain upbeat about your sexual experience. Consider obstacles as opportunities for development and acknowledge your progress. A happy and fulfilled sexual life is greatly influenced by having a positive outlook.

Never forget that having a satisfying sexual life is a lifelong process. Your entire life will be more fulfilling and enriching if you make an investment in your sexual well-being and confront obstacles with openness and perseverance.

Final Assurance of Guaranteed Results

The methods and approaches covered in this guide are based on accepted theories of psychology, holistic health, and sexual health, even though there are no one-size-fits-all answers. Recognizing the unique differences in reactions and experiences is crucial, though. It could take some time, effort, and constant dedication to become proficient at controlling premature ejaculation.

The knowledge that growth is attainable with perseverance and effort, and that this path is valuable, provides comfort. Counseling with therapists, sex educators, or medical experts can offer specific advice to individuals in need of extra help. Recall that pursuing sexual mastery is about appreciating the complexity of personal relationships and accepting constant development rather than reaching perfection.

1. Personalized Nature of Solutions: Acknowledge that individualized tactics are necessary to combat premature ejaculation. What suits one person could not suit another. The commitment to investigating and customizing methods that suit your particular requirements and tastes provides the assurance.

2. Advancement Above Excellence: Making progress rather than reaching perfection is what gives one confidence. A dedication to the effort, tiny triumphs, and constant improvement are the characteristics of successful management of premature ejaculation.

3. Holistic Approach for Lasting Results: Your all-encompassing strategy, which includes communication techniques, mindfulness training, lifestyle modifications, and even expert advice, helps to create long-lasting effects. These components work together to improve your overall sexual health.

4. Flexibility in Varying Situations: Because life is dynamic, things change. Your ability to adjust and grow with these changes will provide you peace of mind. Remain receptive to modifying your strategy in light of fresh perspectives, life events, and the changing dynamics of your intimate relationship.

5. Ongoing Assistance and Education: This guarantee also covers the continuing assistance and education you give yourself. Remain educated, ask for help when you need it, and cultivate an open-minded, growth-oriented mindset. The path to sexual mastery is a lifelong one, and consistent advancement is guaranteed by your dedication.

6. Beneficial Effect on Life Quality: You work outside the bedroom to address early ejaculation. You're improving your general quality of life by placing a high priority on your sexual health. The

advantages spill over into confidence, emotional connection, and a holistic sense of well-being.

In conclusion, even while it might not be possible to provide a timeframe or precise result, you can be confident in the dedication you've demonstrated to your sexual health. Your journey has been a worthwhile investment in yourself, and you will reap the rewards in the form of increased intimacy, better personal development, and a more fulfilling sexual life. Proceed with assurance, understanding that your endeavors much enhance your general pleasure and well-being.